Caring For/Caring About
Women, Home Care and Unpaid Caregiving

Caring For/Caring About

Women, Home Care and Unpaid Caregiving

Edited by

Karen R. Grant
Carol Amaratunga
Pat Armstrong
Madeline Boscoe
Ann Pederson
Kay Willson

*A volume in the **Health Care in Canada Series**.*
General Editor: Pat Armstrong, York University

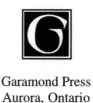

Garamond Press
Aurora, Ontario

Printed and bound in Canada

Garamond Press Ltd,
63 Mahogany Court, Aurora, Ontario L4G 6M8

National Library of Canada Cataloguing in Publication

Caring for/caring about : women, home care, and unpaid caregiving / edited by Karen R. Grant ... [et al.].

(Health care in Canada series)
Includes bibliographical references and index.
ISBN 1-55193-048-X

1. Caregivers—Canada. 2. Women—Employment—Canada.
3. Women—Social conditions. 4. Home care services—Canada.
5. Sexual division of labor—Canada. I. Grant, Karen R. (Karen Ruth), 1957-
II. Series: Health care in Canada (Aurora, Ont.)

RA645.37.C3C37 2004   649.8'0971   C2004-901140-5

This project was financially supported by the Women's Health Contribution Program, Women's Health Bureau, Health Canada. The views expressed herein do not necessarily represent the views or official policy of Health Canada.

Garamond Press gratefully acknowledges the support of the Department of Canadian Heritage, Government of Canada, and the support of the Ontario Media Development Corporation of the Government of Ontario.

Contents

The Health Care in Canada Series
General Editor: Pat Armstrong

Acknowledgements

Many individuals contributed to the production of this book. We are particularly indebted to those who attended the National Think Tank on Women on Unpaid Caregiving in November 2001 and who shared their expertise on how to address research and policy on women, home care and unpaid caregiving. Their insights and analyses reaffirmed that the right to care for those providing care and for those receiving care must acknowledge women's vital role within the system.

The Think Tank would not have been possible without the financial support provided by Health Canada's Women's Health Contribution Program, and the other sponsors including Veterans Affairs, the CIHR Institute of Gender and Health, and the Prince Edward Island Health Research Institute.

We are grateful to all of the contributors, particularly those who persevered through multiple revisions of their work. Finally, we thank Lesley Cameron for her sensitive editing of this work.

Introduction

We typically think of care in personal rather than social terms. Many authors have argued that the organization and delivery of care continues to be based upon the assumption that caring *about* someone naturally leads to caring *for* them (Noddings 1984; Tronto 1993). This way of thinking reinforces current patterns of family caregiving in which women are estimated to comprise nearly 80 percent of those providing unpaid, direct personal care in Canada and are the majority of workers providing paid home care.

Current trends in health care reform in recent years reinforced the vision that care is a "private trouble," rather than a "public issue" (Mills 1959) as the state reduced its investment in care and support for both paid and unpaid caregivers. Recent discussions in Canada, however, suggest that policy makers are beginning to recognize the burden of caregiving on women and are investigating strategies to improve the situation of women and families (Romanow 2002). We hope this book provides support to this counter trend and increases the options for providing care in our society.

This monograph examines care work, both paid and unpaid, and the current conditions for such work. These conditions arise in a context of globalization and changes to the nation state, families and communities, as well as ideological trends and evolving conceptualizations of women, race, culture, sexuality, age and social justice. Closer to home, federal and provincial/territorial policies structure the conditions of care, setting the terms for who provides and who pays for care to whom, where and when. Finally, individual preferences and personal circumstances affect both the possibilities and limits of caring.

This book builds on a National Think Tank on Gender and Unpaid Caregiving held in Charlottetown, Prince Edward Island, in November 2001.[1] The Think Tank brought together academic and community researchers, paid and unpaid caregivers, policy makers and advocates for three days to discuss the gendered nature of caregiving, to hear about research and identify areas for additional investigation and to examine the experiences of caregiving in the current context. That the Think Tank participants were deeply committed to action became evident with the preparation during the final hours of the Think Tank of what came to be called "The Charlottetown Declaration on the Right to Care." This book is a further product of our commitment to action as we, the

National Coordinating Group on Health Care Reform and Women, work to make the effort and concerns of the participants visible to a wider audience.

The National Coordinating Group on Health Care Reform and Women came together in 1998 with representatives from the four federally funded Centres of Excellence for Women's Health, the Canadian Women's Health Network, and the Women's Health Bureau of Health Canada. Our mandate is to coordinate research on health care reform, to identify gaps in research and take steps to fill those gaps, and to translate research into policies and practices. While home and community care have been on the public policy agenda for many years in Canada, the establishment of the Commission on the Future of Health Care in Canada in April 2001 provided a vital opportunity to raise our voices with respect to this pressing issue. We were fortunate to have the opportunity to share the results of the Think Tank, on behalf of the participants, with the Commission in the spring of 2002. In its Final Report (Romanow 2002) the Commission stressed the fact that Canadians want and need a comprehensive health care system that encompasses home and community-based care. Little recognition was given, however, to the fact that care is primarily women's work and women's responsibility.

We hope, therefore, that this book encourages further discussion of the current practices and policies regarding care work, changing trends and possible futures. The book includes all the papers presented during the Think Tank – several of which have been revised and updated – as well as some papers commissioned by the editors, based upon discussions at the Think Tank. For example, participants identified the need for greater visibility and research into home care as it concerns women with disabilities and Aboriginal women. We are pleased to have enlarged this monograph with chapters on both topics. In addition, chapters include an analysis of the historical context of care work in Canada, a companion piece on care in the new millennium, a review of home care research and policy from the perspective of gender, and two papers that discuss how we might design home and community care to serve the needs of people for active citizenship and human dignity.

The overriding question behind this book is: How do we make care possible in the current fiscal, political and social context? Each of the contributions offers us some guidelines that will help make it possible for women to continue to care about others in their lives and to have greater choice in when, where and how to care for them.

Notes

1. Details of the Think Tank are reported in the proceedings, *The Objective is Care: Proceedings of The National Think Tank on Gender and Unpaid Caregiving* (Pederson and Beattie-Huggan 2002) available at http://www.cewh-cesf.ca/healthreform/home_care/index.html

---

References

Mills, C.W. (1959). *The Sociological Imagination*. New York: Oxford University Press.

Noddings, N. (1984). *Caring: A Feminine Approach to Ethics and Moral Education*. Berkeley: University of California Press.

Romanow, R. (2002). *Building on Values: The Future of Health Care in Canada, Final Report*. Ottawa: The Royal Commission on the Future of Health Care in Canada.

Tronto, J. (1993). *Moral Boundaries: A Political Argument for an Ethic of Care*. New York: Routledge.

Thinking It Through:
Women, Work and Caring in the New Millennium

Pat Armstrong and Hugh Armstrong

The U.S. feminist Deborah Stone, an eloquent analyst of women's caring, talks about being a "'lumper' rather than a 'splitter'" (Stone 2000:91). For "lumpers," the emphasis is on what is common about women's work, what women share. At the same time, there remains in her publications a clear recognition of tensions and differences. Miriam Glucksmann's revealing analyses of British women's work speaks of "slicing" data, theory and concepts to create multiple and complex pictures of particular peoples in particular places (Glucksmann 2000:16). Her purpose is to look at the various ways in which work is divided up within what she calls the "total social organization of labour."

This chapter is about both lumping and slicing. It attempts to explore what is common, not only among women but also across time and space. At the same time, it seeks to examine different slices of the same questions. Such slices are meant to help expose the complex and contradictory nature of the concepts we use in considering women's work and of the current state of women's work. It assumes that contexts and locations matter and that, while women face considerable pressures from forces outside their immediate control, they are also active participants in shaping their own lives.

WHY LUMP?

Throughout recorded time, there has been a division of labour by gender. Every known society has not only defined some work as men's and some as women's, they have also distinguished between what women do and do not do. Women have primary daily responsibility for children and for the sick or disabled, as well as for much other domestic work. They do most of the cooking, washing, cleaning, toileting, bathing, feeding, comforting, training for daily living, shopping and planning for domestic consumption and care. And it is women who bear the children. The division of labour is combined with a gap between average male and female wages. Jobs mainly done by men are paid more than those mainly done by women. Women are much more likely than men to work part-time or part-year, and to have interrupted career patterns or casual, temporary jobs. When self-employed, they are much less likely than men to employ others. And much of the work women do is paid no wage at all.

Feminists have long struggled to make the full range of women's work both visible and valued, and lumping allows them to do this. They began in the early 1960s by focusing on domestic labour, understood as the unpaid work women do in households, and by revealing the institutional and social arrangements that combine to produce systemic discrimination in the paid workforce. Initially the emphasis was on what was termed the reproduction of labour power on a daily and generational basis – i.e., having babies and providing for their needs and those of their breadwinning fathers. As the research on women's work expanded, the picture became both more refined and more complex. More categories of work, such as care for the elderly, the sick and the disabled, appeared in the literature. This care category was then also further refined to include care management, assistance with daily living, and personal as well as medical care, and it came to be seen as a relationship rather than simply a work category. Similarly, the picture of women's work in the labour force was further developed to encompass the detailed division of labour found within occupations and industries and the nature of workplace relationships. Within the formal economy outside the home, working in the public sector was distinguished from the private sector, and then this private sector itself was divided between the for-profit and the not-for-profit, or what came to be called the third sector. Within the not-for-profit sector, women's work as volunteers was distinguished from their paid employment, and their role in the underground economy, where they worked for pay as cleaners, prostitutes, babysitters and secretaries, and in formal economy jobs that they did in their own homes, was also revealed.

Lumping also allows us to explore the social, economic and institutional arrangements as well as the policies and practices that contribute to these patterns in women's work. But lumping is not only about processes remote from the individual lives of most women, about abstract concepts or far-away decision-makers. It is also about how women's work is shaped at the level of the hospital, day care, community centre, clinic, home and office, about the fine divisions of labour, the ways policies are played out in daily lives and the ways women act to create spaces in their own lives or to limit those spaces. So, for example, lumping allows us to ask what kinds of caring work women and men do, and what kinds of government funding support or undermine this work.

Lumping, then, is appropriate because there are so many common patterns in women's work. Lumping allows us to see what women, as women, share, in terms of the nature of both the work and the work relationships. It also helps us to expose the forces that keep these patterns in place and change them.

WHY SLICE?

Although there is a division of labour by gender everywhere, there is no common division of labour across time and space, often not even within countries during a particular period. What is defined and practiced as men's work or women's work varies enormously and most cultures have at least some women who do men's work. Moreover, the actual division of labour can contradict the prescriptions or accepted practices. Equally important, among women there are significant differences related to class, race, culture, age, marital status, sexual orientation and spatial locations, as well as for the same women over time.

The range of forms this division can take, if not a comprehensive listing of them, is illustrated by the following. Once those paid to do secretarial and teaching work were mainly men, now most are women. Those paid as chefs are mainly men, while women do most of the unpaid cooking. However, in Canada at least, if the unpaid cooking is done outside on the barbecue, it is men who do the work but the unpaid kitchen jobs are still primarily left to women. In the former USSR, most doctors were women at the same time as North American medicine was dominated by men. The care provided by women in a Bosnian refugee camp differs fundamentally from that provided in a household in Ottawa's exclusive Rockcliffe neighbourhood. While care work is women's work, there are multiple forms of women's paid and unpaid caring. There are also considerable variations across time and place as to what is defined as women's caring work. Our grandmothers, for example, did not clean catheters, insert needles or adjust oxygen masks as part of the care work they did at home.

In addition, large gaps may show in both places between what women and men think they should do and what they are able to do. There is, in other words, often a gap between practices and ideas about appropriate practices. For example, while most Canadian and British men seem to think they should equally share the domestic labour, there is little evidence that such sharing actually happens in practice. Many men who think care is women's work find themselves providing care for ill and aging partners; many women who provide care do not necessarily think that it is their job, nor do they necessarily have the skills to do the work. At the same time, many women who think they should provide care cannot do so because they have too many other demands on their time, because they do not have the skills, because they do not have the other necessary resources or because they do not have the physical capacity. Many who do provide care – providing services such as meal preparation, comforting and cleaning – may not even see this as care because it is so much a part of their daily lives.

There may also be significant differences among women within workplaces. A hospital, for example, may have women working as managers and as housekeepers. The managers are more likely to be white, Canadian-born, with English or French as a first language, and relatively young, while the housekeepers are more likely to have migrated to this country, to have neither English or French as their mother tongue and to be older than the female managers. And, of course, there are significant differences between these groups in terms of power, pay and ideas about work, and in their political, material and symbolic resources related not only to their positions in the paid workforce but also to their positions in their households and neighbourhoods.

However, slicing does more than draw out the differences related to women's various spatial, physical, social, psychological, economic, work and age locations. It is necessary in order to see the different ways of understanding and developing the evidence and different views on the same processes. It is, for example, possible to look at care from the perspective of the care provider or from that of those with care needs, or to examine care as a relationship. Furthermore, the family as a group may see care issues one way; the government, the agencies and the paid providers in other ways. Indeed, each household member may have a specific way of slicing the situation. Equally important, the tensions among these may not be possible to resolve but only to recognize and handle. By beginning with a recognition of contradiction, by taking this slice it is possible to develop policies and practices that seek to accommodate such tensions, rather than setting out single solutions based on notions of harmony.

Analysis can begin from a number of different questions – for example, what does this mean in the short term and what does it mean in the long term? What does it mean for those immediately involved and what does it mean for the country or the world? It can also begin by acknowledging that some practices, conditions and situations are contradictory. Women, for example, may simultaneously want to provide care but find it impossible to do so. They may love the person for whom they provide care but, precisely because of this love, dislike providing care.

Slicing can expose the different kinds of care work involved in providing for children with and without disabilities; for teenagers who join gangs and for those unable to attend university because there is no money; for adult neighbours with chronic illness and for those with marital problems; for healthy seniors and severely ill seniors. It can also reveal what it means to provide this care at home or in an institution, and what different kinds of institutions and homes there are.

The initial purposes can be quite varied. For example, most policies are about helping households and families adapt to the demands of paid work and services. As some Norwegian policy analysts make clear, we can also start by figuring out how paid work can adapt to family lives (Brandth and Kvande 2001). Instead of asking what resources the growing number of elderly require, the questions could be about the resources they bring and the services they provide. Rather than asking how care can be made into an individual responsibility, we can ask what conditions make it possible to care without conscripting women into caregiving. Rather than assuming, as we do in Canada, that public care is what supplements family care done mainly by women, we could assume that families supplement public care.

Slicing adds both a recognition of difference and the possibility of developing different views of the same issues, circumstances and evidence.

WHY WOMEN?

On the one hand, we have a universal pattern in terms of a division of labour by sex and women embracing caring work. On the other hand, we have an incredible range of labour done by women and defined as women's work. We also have women resisting caring work. Indeed, the U.S. historian Emily Abel argues that some nineteenth-century women "complained bitterly that caregiving confined them to the home, caused serious physical and emotional health problems, and added to domestic labour, which was gruelling even in the best of times" (Abel 2000:8). What factors, ideas, structures, and processes contribute to this universality and difference, this embracing and resistance? More specifically, why do women provide the care but in so many different ways? There are no simple answers to these questions, but there are a number of answers that help contribute to a better understanding of care as women's responsibility.

Natural Care Providers?

We know that only women have babies. We also know that the meaning, experience and consequences of having babies varies enormously not only across time, location and culture, but also for individual women and from one baby to another. Céline Dion's experience of giving birth will be fundamentally different from that of an Aboriginal woman who must leave her northern Quebec community to receive medical assistance. Moreover, there is no intrinsic connection between having babies and rearing them; that is, providing care. Bodies are a factor in all of women's lives but these bodies are embedded in social, economic and political structures that continually influence how bodies work, as well as how they are defined and valued. They cannot explain why women provide most of the care not only for the babies they bear but for other people as well.

Although there is plenty of evidence to suggest that women are more likely than men to identify with the emotional aspects of caring, there is very little evidence to suggest that this is connected to the way women's bodies or minds are physiologically constructed or that men are physiologically incapable of such caring emotions. On the contrary, there is evidence to suggest that girls are taught, and expected to exhibit, such caring and that they are also more likely than their brothers to be assigned the caring jobs in the home. What sociologists call early socialization obviously contributes to women's skills in and attitudes to care, as well as to their brothers' notions of who is responsible for and able to care. However, the pressures on women to provide care do not end with, and perhaps are not even primarily created by, early learning. Just as children are born and formed within a social context, so too are women carers daily created and shaped within social relationships, processes, and structures. At the same time, women are active in creating these same relationships, processes and structures, albeit often from a weaker position than that of men.

These relationships, processes and structures are about power, not only in the sense that governments, employers, community organizations and husbands have specific powers and protect specific rights but also in the more general sense of whose preferences, ways of acting and ideas prevail in daily practices. And they are about resources – the principles as well as the mechanisms for their distribution. Power and resources in the formal and underground economies, in community organizations and households, are often mutually reinforcing and are definitely linked. They are also unequally distributed, not only between women and men but also among women. Women do have resources and are active participants in creating caring work. However, most women have fewer resources than most men do and the resources that they do have, as well as the means of participating, are frequently different from those of men.

There is, then, very little that is "natural" about women's work in general or their caring work in particular. Contexts matter much more than bodies in creating and maintaining women's caring work. Caring can be understood as women's work only within the unequal relationships, structures and processes that help create women as carers and undervalue this caring work.

THINKING GLOBALLY: THE LARGEST CONTEXT

Globalization has become a familiar term in recent years. However, teasing out its meanings and its implications for women in different locations is a complicated task. Globalization implies a process that is drawing the world and its occupants closer together, on what is often seen as an inevitable and undirected path. At the core of this process are giant corporations centred in one, usually Northern, country but operating throughout the globe. These transnational corporations (TNCs) helped create the technologies that have themselves contributed both to the corporations' multinational form and their power. Such technologies make it possible to move money rapidly around the globe to avoid, or at least threaten to avoid, any particular government's taxes and regulations by moving their investments. They also make it possible to move work around the world, thus allowing the corporations to avoid, or threaten to avoid, demands from workers or restrictions on the use of labour imposed by governments. In order to facilitate this movement of goods, money and work, the giant corporations have been central in promoting what is often called free trade. Free trade is far from new, and traders have always enjoyed considerable freedoms and power, but it may well be that the speed of transactions has altered along with the size of the corporations directing them. As a result, their power may be greater than ever before.

Instead of combining to resist the pressure from TNCs, many governments have come together to support the process of achieving greater and easier movement of goods, services and money. At the international level, the First World countries (also called Northern, developed or industrial countries) in particular have worked through the International Monetary Fund, the World Bank and the World Trade Organization to promote the removal of restrictions on trade, a process that entails both deregulation and re-regulation. Countries with enormous debts have been required to introduce structural adjustment programs that involve the removal of many restrictions on foreign investment and labour practices, as well as the sale of public corporations to private ones, cutbacks in public services and the adoption of market strategies within the public sector that remains. The impact on women has been mixed and contradictory, both within and across nations.

Women from all over the world have found new jobs on the "global assembly line," producing goods and even services previously produced mainly by women in the highly industrialized countries. Companies have relocated to other countries to avoid high wages and restrictions on working conditions so the jobs for women have rarely been good ones. But they have offered some new possibilities for work, income, shared locations and minimal protections. More common has been the expansion of paid work for women outside the factory walls within the underground or informal economy where few, if any, rules apply. Women have been drawn into small-scale retail and service work, into domestic and home-work or simply into semi-clandestine enterprises (Ward 1990). Here the boundaries between household and formal economy, between public and private space, and between employment time and non-employment time are blurred, and protection, along with visibility, is absent. At the same time, the withdrawal of public services has meant that women have had to do more of this work without pay or support within the confines of their private worlds where the work is less visible and less available. For many women within these countries, there is no paid work at all. The poverty and unemployment that follow in the wake of structural adjustment policies push many to search for jobs in those First World countries that have created these policies. Women in particular have sought work as what Grace Chang calls "disposable domestics" (Chang 2000). Separated in time and space from their children, these women often do the domestic and caring work for First World women under conditions supported in the First World by the combination of government regulations, women's working conditions and the failure to provide care services. Like free trade, the movement of women to do such work is not new but the scale has altered. The result is a growing gap among women within and between countries, a gap that is also frequently linked to racialized categories.

In addition to imposing structural adjustment programs on Third World countries (or what are often called Southern or developing countries) First World countries have entered into trade agreements that promise to support the movement of goods, services, money and, to a lesser extent, people across borders. This has not necessarily meant less government, but it has meant more measures to allow corporations to operate with less regard to national practices and preferences and fewer taxes or other contributions to national economies. It has also meant less local and democratic control as more decisions are made by these international trading groups. Facing debt pressures themselves, these countries have adopted strategies similar to those imposed on the Third World. First World countries have acted more like entrepreneurs at the same time as they have handed over more of the services previously provided by governments to private, for-profit firms.

These shifts have had critical consequences for women. The expansion of the public sector had provided many, and often quite good, jobs for women. Indeed, "in 1981, between 65 and 75 percent of college-educated women in Germany, Sweden and the USA were employed in the 'social welfare industries'" (Pierson 1999:130). Many of these jobs disappeared, or their character changed, in the wake of the global reforms. Trade agreements allowed some women to move to other countries in search of work – registered nurses, for example, left Canada in large numbers when hospitals closed, to find jobs in the United States – but those women from Third World countries seeking work in Canada found it more difficult to gain full citizenship status, providing just one example of how free trade has not worked in the same way for everyone.

As public services have declined, more of the services have been provided for sale in the market. This process, often described as commodification, determines access primarily on the ability to pay rather than on need. More women in First World countries than in Third World have had the means to pay for commodified services. However, women in both Worlds have continued to earn less than men and continued to bear primary responsibility for care and domestic work. Faced with public fewer services and relatively low pay, but still in need of income to purchase the services, women in the First World have sought the cheapest means of paying for care or other supports. This often involves the even poorer women from the Third World. This is not to suggest that most First World women have completely escaped unpaid work or that the majority of women could afford to pay for services. Indeed the reduction in public services has meant that a considerable amount of this work formerly done by women for pay in the market is now done by women without pay in the home. In other words, it has been decommodified but not eliminated. Rather, the point is that just as globalization creates and reinforces linkages among women, so also these linkages create and reinforce divisions among them.

Globalization does not simply refer to economics, however. It also refers to the ways in which people, ideas and cultures are brought closer together around the world. This has, in many ways, meant the spread of First World, and especially U.S., practices. Along with music, movies, fashions and food have come ideas about all aspects of social life, including women's work. This dissemination of ideas is also linked in many ways to the corporations, both through their ownership of companies that produce these goods and through their influence over the media. In these global sources, the emphasis is increasingly on the individual as a consumer with choices based on the capacity to purchase. Like the relocation of jobs, the spread of ideas is a mixed blessing. On the one hand, feminist ideas have spread rapidly around the world. On the other hand, it is the First World version of feminism that has spread most rapidly and this version too often fails to take into account context and difference.

The notion of shared international perspectives is not particularly new. Indeed, after World War II there was much talk of a postwar consensus based on a commitment to expanded government-provided services, a mixed economy that combined public and private enterprise, and policies of full employment along with sustained economic growth (Pierson 1999:125). Redistribution of goods and services was part of the package, as were collective responsibility and shared risk. This consensus seems to have fallen apart, replaced by a new, and quite different, one. Public rights are replaced by private ones, with markets rather than states as the preferred means of allocating jobs, goods and services. But markets are unable to respond to many human needs and are especially ill-equipped to promote equity and full employment, or to avoid long-term problems like pollution or other health consequences. They actually result in greater inequality, especially for women. As the British theorist Ian Gough explains, "Markets paradoxically require altruistic, collective behaviour on the part of women in the household in order to enable men to act individualistically in the market" (Gough 2000:16).

Globalization has allowed much more than money, people, goods and services to move quickly around the world. Diseases too face more permeable borders. New epidemics such as HIV/AIDS and old ones like tuberculosis and hepatitis are transported around the globe with relative ease, transported in and by airplanes and service workers. Increasing inequality, not only in the Third World but also in the First, encourages the development of these diseases and prevents their treatment. Diabetes has become much more common, especially among marginalized groups in large urban centres and on reservations. With an incidence rate, conservatively estimated, at two to three times that of non-Aboriginal peoples, the National Forum on Health termed diabetes among Aboriginal peoples a "growing pandemic" (National Forum on Health 1997:6). At the same time, protections under free trade rules for pharmaceutical patents frequently leave treatments beyond the reach of many.

One way, then, to slice globalization is to reveal the increasing dominance of transnational corporations, the converging of governments around market strategies, the declining democratic controls and the growing gap for and among women. Another way is to expose the counter tendencies. The same technologies that support corporate power allow various kinds of social and labour movements to organize around their interests. We see evidence of this not only in the "battle of Seattle" and in the streets of Quebec, but also in the Beijing Conference on Women that reached a consensus around means of promoting women's equality and in the attempts to protect sweatshop workers encouraged by the success of Naomi Klein's book *No Logo* (Klein 2000). The movement of people around the globe has meant that many of us are now more familiar with other cultures and practices.

We also see counter tendencies in the escalation, and power, of terrorism. Although many governments have adopted strategies taken from the for-profit sector, there is still an incredible variety in the ways these governments operate. Many countries retain important public programs that reflect a continuing commitment to social rights and collective responsibility. Others have taken a route that emphasizes family values while still others have turned to religion and ethnicity. Moreover, the trade alliance among members of the European Union has served to improve working conditions for many women and help improve services for others. Instead of deregulation we see on occasion the extension of regulation. The U.K., for example, has been required to provide protections for part-time workers and to introduce both minimum wage and equal pay legislation, all of which improve women's market jobs. Several countries are resisting the high drug prices that prevent them from treating mothers with HIV/AIDS, a sign that not all countries are willing to put property rights above people's right to life. And, perhaps most importantly, there is ample evidence to demonstrate that spending on social programs can enhance rather than prevent trade and that gender-based analysis linked to effective programs is essential to economic development.

Contradictions within global developments, as well as those among particular kinds of developments, are important in understanding where and how change may occur or is occurring. It is equally important to examine the details of how global agreements and patterns are played out within specific locations, because practices may well defy or transform intentions.

In short, globalization is about processes that result from actual decisions and practices rather than about forces beyond human control. While there is strong evidence to demonstrate that corporations are powerful players often supported by governments, there is also evidence to suggest that there are both limits on this power and contradictory patterns. There are choices to be made, choices that can have important consequences for women and their work, and have to be considered in developing strategies for care.

THINKING NATIONALLY: THE CANADIAN STATE

The debates around globalization have led to questions about the power of the nation state, while the emphasis on markets has led to talk about the end of the welfare state. The state in these debates refers to much more than government in the narrow sense of elected officials, the legal system and the bureaucracy that supports them. It also refers to more than the right to rule over a specific territory. While it certainly involves these well-known aspects, it also includes the broad range of institutions, policies, practices and relations that together constitute governance.

Those who talk about the end of the nation state base their claims on the rise of global corporations and development of both international agreements and international institutions. Globalization from this perspective means the demise of national sovereignty. Some fear this decline, arguing that it means nations can no longer make their own choices and that democratic control is undermined. Health care is a case in point. Although the current Canadian government argues that national, public health care is protected under a special clause in the North American Free Trade Agreement (NAFTA), legal opinions sought by union and other groups warn that the public system is quite vulnerable to foreign investment and thus foreign control under this Agreement. Nations have clearly surrendered some rights in signing these agreements and give away even more perhaps in negotiating separately with corporations and in creating the conditions for foreign investment. However, as Dexter Whitfield puts it in his book on this issue, "the nation state continues to play a crucial role in creating and maintaining the conditions for capital accumulation, ensuring the health, education and safety of citizens, providing a framework for social relations, and maintaining civil society" (Whitfield 2001:18-19). Undoubtedly, Canadians still have important powers in terms of establishing the conditions for work and in deciding how, when and where care is provided, even though both federal and provincial governments have surrendered some powers to corporations and global decision-making organizations.

The Changing Welfare State

Those who talk about the end of the welfare state point to the "shrinking" of the public sector (Shields and Evans 1998) as well as to a shift away from a notion of collective rights and responsibilities along with the adoption of market strategies. Welfare is, of course, not new. States were involved in welfare programs long before World War II. Canadian governments supported hospitals and schools, charitable organizations and widowed mothers through allowances, for example. But World War II marked a qualitative change in the guiding philosophy, and in the extent as well as the nature of state intervention. The period from that war's end until the mid-1970s has become known as the "Golden Years" of the welfare state because they were not only the years of the most comprehensive and universal social programs, they were also marked by a notion of shared risk and collective rights that meant the state bore overall responsibility for the welfare of citizens and for limiting the negative impact of markets. States played a more active and visible role in the redistribution of income, power and other resources, and in the delivery of services. Any redistribution from those with these resources to those without is likely to benefit women more than men because women have fewer resources than men do. These developments both reflected and contributed to postwar prosperity, and were linked directly to the demands from unions, citizen organizations and women's groups for a better world.

During this postwar period, Canada introduced universal family allowances and pensions, paid to everyone in the maternal and old age categories as a right of citizenship. Pensions meant that many women in particular escaped poverty and could live independently in their old age. Universal health coverage for necessary doctor and hospital care also proved to help poor women significantly and without the stigma of a means tests. This meant not only that all Canadians had the right to health care as a right of citizenship, but that they had more choices about publicly provided care and that there was no need to sort the deserving from the undeserving. Education was also provided on a universal basis, allowing many more women to continue beyond elementary school. However, tuition fees remained at the post-secondary level and thus still constituted a barrier for many seeking to become experts in care. Additional barriers linked to race, culture and other locations also remained because the main focus was on ensuring the same access, rather than on recognizing and accommodating differences. Universal treatment can mean treatment based on a standard that assumes everyone has the same needs, and too often that standard is a white, relatively healthy and wealthy male. Welfare, child care, home care and long-term care received significantly more resources, but they remained means-tested services directed at those who could prove they were deserving. Although women's position at home and in the labour force meant they were more likely than men to fit these criteria, the construction of these programs often served to reinforce, rather than alleviate, women's dependency.

Immigration rules were changed in an attempt to make Canada more open to people from a broader range of countries with a wider range of backgrounds. As a result, Canada became a much more racially and culturally mixed society. However, supports were still lacking, especially for the women who came as dependents. And there were still important barriers, such as those that applied to the recognitions of foreign credentials for nurses or other professionals and those that applied to women entering as domestics. Racism remained embedded in most social and economic structures and relationships, but many more immigrants were nonetheless able to enter and thrive. Aboriginal peoples may have fared less well than immigrants and Aboriginal women certainly fared less well than all other women in terms of jobs, pay and protections. Perhaps the best that can be said of this period is that there was a movement away from a policy of assimilation towards one of recognition, after hard struggles by Aboriginal peoples against state initiatives.

Canada also intervened directly in the market to introduce employment protections that influenced the distribution of power. Labour standards legislation provided for a minimum wage and improvements in some health and safety regulations, along with other rights such as statutory holidays and overtime regulations. These changes were much more likely to protect the women who fill the majority of the lowest paid and least unionized labour force jobs, many of which involve providing care. The same was true of human rights legislation. Meanwhile, unemployment insurance and workers' compensation were intended to provide income for workers whose jobs disappeared or who were injured at work. Both programs recognized that job loss was often the fault of employers or the economy, rather than individual workers, but the way they were structured and implemented meant they applied mainly to men. The same was true for the workplace-linked Canada/Quebec pension scheme. Moreover, the regulations and benefits seldom applied to part-time, short-term or casual work where women were found in far greater numbers than men and where work often involved care. Full employment policies were more frequently preached than practiced but, to the extent that they contributed to higher employment levels, they did help to redistribute income.

State investment in these health, education and welfare programs meant enormous job expansion in the public sector. Many of these jobs went to women because women were available, they needed the income, they had the training and the work was clearly defined as women's work. By the end of the "Golden Years," almost one in three employed women worked in the broader public sector. Brought together in large work places, women formed unions and demanded the state live up to its international commitments to equality. As a result, the state not only provided benefits, services and protections; it also provided jobs, many of which were quite good jobs in terms of pay, benefits and security. A majority of the jobs were about providing care in one form or another. With pay came some recognition that care is work, and that care requires some support and training. Women's pay and better access to higher education also helped increase their power within households, as did new rules on property rights, violence and abuse.

The impact of the welfare state in these years was contradictory and far from perfect for women, or for particular groups of women. Feminists have rightly criticized the welfare state for failing to substantially reduce inequality between women and men or among women. They have argued that, in many ways, the rise of the welfare state meant that rule by the father or husband was replaced with rule by the state, and that many programs and policies have served to reinforce women's segregation in the labour force and responsibility for care inside and outside the formal economy. They have objected to the bureaucratic rules and institutional practices that standardized care in ways that eliminated the personal, the dominance of professionals who failed to take women's needs into account, and the failure to support women's independence from families or the state.

At the same time, the welfare state did improve the lot of many women. Some income was redistributed from the rich to the poor and from men to women. Services funded by the state were even more successful at improving access for women and so were many of the protections against employers and spouses provided by the state. Professional autonomy meant practitioners could base decisions on individual cases, and government benefits, along with programs and services, did allow some women to make choices about their private lives. Moreover, it was much easier for women to influence the state than to influence employers, given access to some democratic means of participation in the state sector. Consequently, women still looked first to the state for an expansion of rights and care.

Since the mid-1970s, there has been a fundamental transformation in guiding philosophies and actual state practices. There has been a slow but steady shift away from the notion of shared risk to one of individual risk and responsibility, from social rights to individual consumer rights. Instead of a commitment to full employment through state intervention, there has been a growing commitment to reliance on market mechanisms in and outside the state, as well as an emphasis on individual responsibility for finding and keeping paid work. State initiatives are designed more to support the market than to limit its impact. Markets, rather than states, are to be the main mechanism for redistribution. On the basis of arguments about both debt loads and poor public sector practices, public programs and protections have been reduced. Fees have been added and services cut back. New regulations have been introduced to sort the deserving from the undeserving and to limit the power of unions. Services have been privatized or had private sector techniques applied. In the process, many of women's good jobs in the public sector have been eliminated or transformed while less of the caring work is provided with little or no charge in the public sector. Care still needs to be done, but less is done for pay in the public sector or provided without direct financial cost to citizens. While the number of public employees has shrunk, the power of the state within Canada has not.

The elimination of the deficit and the reduction of the debt have made it more difficult to use these as the basis for reform, but the state continues to pursue market-oriented ideas and practices. They now tend to be justified on the basis of the growing number of the elderly and the rising expectations of "consumers," most of whom are women. Yet there is increasing evidence to show that there is no inevitable increase in dependency with aging. As the British authors in a recent book on aging put it, "the association of aging with disease and inevitable decline is better reframed so that aging is seen as a *social* rather than *biological process*" (Estes et al. 2001:31). There is also evidence to show that the very market mechanisms designed to save public investment in care promote the same rising expectations that are defined as the problem.

Governments at the federal and provincial levels have simultaneously decentralized some responsibilities while centralizing other powers. Decentralization has been promoted as a means of enhancing local decision-making, but it has been combined with a reduction in resources and often increased regulations about what local authorities can do and how they should do it. As a result, local decision-makers may be left with the responsibility for cuts but not the choices about whether or how to cut. This may mean they are pushed to privatization, both in keeping with government regulations and in an effort to deal with costs in the short term. Moreover, groups such as lesbians and Aboriginal peoples may find it difficult to have their voices heard at the local level because their numbers are small.

One obvious result of these developments, established by various research projects, is the existence of growing gaps among people (see, for example, Yalnizyan 1998). Income gaps are growing between women and men and among women in ways linked to race and other locations. While the "Golden Years" of the welfare state did not create equality, they did reduce inequality and their end is marked by new patterns of inequality and the reinforcement of old ones. There are increasing gaps in power as well as in income, and there are increasing symbolic gaps as well. For example, women on welfare and women who use emergency rooms are increasingly defined as abusers of the system, and women's groups are described as protecting "special interests" (see, for example, Little 2001; Cardozo 1996).

Nevertheless, some important services, benefits and protections remain. Hospital and doctor care provide the best examples. The continued existence of a universal health care scheme, albeit one in the process of reforms that may transform it, is testimony to both the power of citizen support and the effectiveness of the program in providing care. Some commitment to collective rights and responsibility clearly remains. Moreover, some supports like shelters for battered women have been restored or expanded, also in response to citizen claims. Some pensions are still universal. Important rights, like those protected by the *Charter of Rights and Freedoms* and the *Canadian Human Rights Act,* have been maintained. There are also significant differences among jurisdictions in Canada, demonstrating both that there are still choices to be made and that citizens' protests can still make a difference.

These state practices set the context for care. In providing supports, benefits, services and regulations, or in not providing these, states establish the conditions for care in and outside the formal economy. The state plays a fundamental role in determining how political, material and symbolic resources are distributed and in mediating the distribution of these among markets, communities, households and individuals. Indeed, states are central in determining what is public and what is private in the formal economy and what is private in the sense of being outside the formal economy. The benefits and negative consequences are unevenly distributed between women and men and among women. It is thus necessary not only to find out what the state does, but also to determine who benefits and how they benefit, if we are to figure out how to create good conditions for care.

THINKING MARKETS: INVISIBLE AND VISIBLE HANDS

While the welfare state has not disappeared, the role it plays in relation to the market has changed in terms of both policy statements and policy practices. This is not to suggest that the market was not strongly supported by the state even in the "Golden Years," but rather to indicate the new and public emphasis on markets as the best means of both delivering and distributing services. Once defined as public goods largely produced and distributed outside the market, care services are increasingly defined as market goods to be produced by for-profit means and distributed according to consumer preferences. Market mechanisms are assumed to be more efficient at producing services because producers want to both create the best services possible in order to attract customers and spend less in order to ensure profits. Thus the search for profit, combined with competition in an open market where everyone has equal opportunity, leads an "invisible hand" to develop the best services at the best price through the best means.

There are several problems with these assumptions, especially as they apply to care. First, markets have never been free in the sense implied by the notions of an open market with equal opportunities and no directing hands. States actively protect property rights, for example, in ways that directly contradict this notion and, in the process, favour some market participants over others. So pharmaceutical companies can patent products for twenty or more years to protect them from competition and can deduct expenditures on research and development from their taxable income. In the process, the public assumes much of the risk that is invoked by these companies as justification for their patent protections and their huge profits.

Second, there is a tendency towards monopoly as companies seek to buy out the competition, in the process eliminating much of the very competition that is supposed to be the essence of the market. Again, this process is abetted by the state. To return to the pharmaceutical sector, much of the research and development expenditure that its firms deduct from taxable income are in reality marketing initiatives that actually reduce and eliminate competition. Third, the market is riddled with "irrational" processes that prevent the kind of allocation that the notion of an invisible hand implies. Systemic discrimination in job allocation, for example, contradicts the equal opportunities claim.

Fourth, consumers have fundamentally unequal power when they come to the market as purchasers. The inequalities are not simply about money; they are also about information, access and time. These inequalities are then perpetuated and magnified by market mechanisms that mean that certain choices prevail. Fifth, there is little firm evidence to show that the companies producing the best products in the best way even survive. States cannot afford to let many giant companies disappear, even if they are inefficient producers which fail to produce desired goods in the market.

In care services, there are even more problems with the assumptions about market efficacy. First, services are often required on an urgent or emergency basis, leaving no time for comparative shopping. People cannot easily know what illnesses they will get or what services they will require even on a non-urgent basis, with similar implications for comparative shopping. Second, the consequences may be literally fatal or last throughout life. While purchasing the wrong cereal may put off your whole day, failing to buy cancer care could mean death, and the wrong day care can risk your child's current safety or future possibilities. Third, those using the services typically lack the kind of knowledge necessary to make informed choices on complex matters. This is one reason why many who work in care are termed professionals and are accorded the right and responsibility to make choices on our behalf. We do not want these choices made primarily on the basis of cost or profit, as they are in the for-profit system. Fourth, it is difficult to provide continuity in care across services if they are each competing with the others and are owned by for-profit firms that treat information as trade secrets essential to competition. Care services require significant coordination and long-term planning, neither of which is consistent with the market distribution of services. Moreover, competition means some firms disappear, leaving people without their services or with different services. Or it means states step in to support them or take them over, contradicting the very notions basic to market claims.

Fifth, the tendency or even the requirement for monopolies in highly technological services reduces the possibilities for competition. The complexity of health care and the interdependency of its many components, involving skills among a wide range of providers and expensive facilities, means that integrated care can be delivered by only a few organizations, reducing the possibilities for the very competition that is needed to produce the most efficient and effective care. In rural communities the populations are too small to support competition among services and, in services such as child care, the profit possibilities too small in most areas to attract for-profit providers. Sixth, consumer purchasing means unequal purchasing because market power is based on resources and thus necessarily perpetuates inequality between women and men as well as among women.

Seventh, the search for profit leads to making providers work as hard as possible and to providing as little care as possible while encouraging people to use as many services as possible, because profits are made by selling more and spending less. It also leads to an emphasis on the care that brings the most economic return, to the neglect of those people or services that cannot bring much or any profit. What is not profitable or not defined as part of care work will be left to individuals or charitable organizations to provide, meaning this care is often left to unpaid providers. Finally, the trust that not only makes the entire system work together but is necessary between care recipient and care provider takes years to produce. It cannot be easily captured or replaced by contractual, market language. And for-profit techniques often undermine the trust among providers within the system as their work is more carefully monitored and controlled.

All these problems apply to market mechanisms inside and outside the public sector. Governments have recognized at least some of them, and have addressed the ones they recognize by introducing "managed competition." This simply means that governments more carefully regulate the way markets in care operate, but it fails to address most of the problems of market mechanisms. And managed competition does nothing to address the problem of applying for-profit techniques within care services.

In short, the market mechanisms that have become so popular with governments have to be carefully scrutinized for their impact on the nature and distribution of both care and care work. There is every reason to believe they will change for the worse who gets what kind of care through paid services and the conditions under which providers work, while increasing inequality and sending more care to communities.

COMMUNITIES

Much reform in public care has been justified in terms of both cost-cutting and efficiency. But it has also been done in the name of sending care closer to home, to communities that are assumed to provide more of the kinds of social and emotional support that research tells us is so central to care. Communities are portrayed as warm, friendly, welcoming places, where everybody knows your name. In the 1960s, these communities were presented as alternatives to impersonal institutions but in the new millennium they are understood as substitutes for public services. Yet it remains unclear exactly what is meant by "communities." There are at least four possible aspects of what constitutes a community.

First, there are the voluntary, religious and charitable communities operating as nonprofit entities. Often organized at the national or international level and called Non-Governmental Organizations (or NGOs) these usually have a local presence. Their care services cover a wide range, although they frequently target particular populations based on the care required, such as those with

HIV/AIDS, those suffering from abuse and those needing palliative care, or based on affiliations such as membership in a church or seniors' group. There were once many local, community hospitals operated by NGOs, but many of them have been eliminated or transformed through restructuring. NGOs are not necessarily small, locally controlled or oriented to collective values, however. The Catholic Church, for example, may operate a local long-term care facility based on decisions made far away. Similarly, its refusal to offer birth control or other reproductive health services in its hospitals reflects a policy determined centrally, not locally.

Many of these organizations have long provided services while others have served as incubators and demonstration projects for new services later taken up by the state. Many also performed an advocacy role and most have received government funding of some sort. With the downloading of services, these community organizations are expected to take on much larger, and often different, loads and any hope of governments adopting demonstrably good services have all but disappeared. So too has the time to advocate as service demands take all the resources. Moreover, the conversion within the state to for-profit practices has meant that these organizations now have to follow similar practices in order to be eligible for funding. Some have to enter competitive bidding processes that also absorb time and money while making jobs even less secure. Women tend to provide the majority of care in these organizations, although they much less often comprise the majority of the decision-makers. Much of the care is unpaid and, when there is pay, it tends to be low, with high job insecurity and no benefits. With the majority of women in the labour force, and there because they need the income, there are few remaining women available to provide the care as volunteers. A growing number of women are not available as volunteers because they are providing the care for others at home. They may also be reluctant to take the paid jobs available in these community organizations, given the wages and benefit structures.

Second, there are for-profit concerns operating at the community level. Extendicare, for example, has the contract for many long-term facilities. Other, foreign-owned, corporations have entered the long-term care facility and home care "market" created by new managed competition strategies introduced by governments or left open by the government's failure to provide public care. Such organizations are neither small nor locally controlled, and their emphasis is at least as much on the search for profit as it is on responding to local needs. In the for-profit sector, pay is usually significantly lower than the pay in public hospitals. Indeed, one of the justifications for the movement of care out of hospitals is the lower cost of long-term care. The costs are lower in large measure because people are paid low or no wages. Yet restructuring of hospitals has meant that many of the same patients with the same needs who used to be cared for in the hospitals are now provided for through these community services.

Third, there are neighbours, friends and extended family members. These communities are based on reciprocal relationships that require time to nurture and support. In order to help each other, they need time. And while they may provide help without intent of gaining any return, the community cannot be sustained over time if there are only those who need care and few who can return the favour. As care demands increase, and fewer women are around to provide care, these reciprocal relationships may well be undermined.

Alongside these various kinds of community, there are families. The concept of family is often more fuzzy than that of community, but it is clear that we often mean family when we refer to community care. Indeed, this fourth kind of community is where most care ends up when care is sent to the "community." Including families under the concept of community may hide their multiple and varied responsibilities. Considering them as part of communities may also hide the quite different logics at work within families, where love, blood and interdependency is assumed to be the glue that keeps this form of community together and that drives people to care. So it perhaps makes more sense to consider families as a separate category. However, they are included here as part of community precisely because they provide the bulk of what is meant by community care.

Like the term community in general, families are pictured as warm, supportive environments that can and want to care. Or if they do not, they should. Families are also usually pictured as being based on a happily married, heterosexual couple with several healthy children and loving grandparents hovering around the edges, sharing and caring for each other.

Some families do fit this vision, but a number of important features are missing from the picture. Most families have only a few members, many with only a mother and her children. These households have no men to share in care, few others to provide support and very limited economic or symbolic resources. A significant number of households are reconstructed from families of previously married spouses who may bring with them multiple caring responsibilities but few resources. Some are based on homosexual relationships in couples who face barriers in accessing care based on notions of heterosexual relationships. Families often live far from their relatives and even from their cultural communities. They may even be isolated from their neighbours by physical distance, culture, resources or time. Most women are in the labour force, primarily because they and their families need the income. Many teenagers too have paid work, often because it is critical to their needs or to those of their families. Many families live below the poverty line and often juggle several jobs even to stay close to it, leaving them with few resources in terms of time, power, social relationships or income. As more members have paid jobs and paid work not only takes more time but also takes up more time at home, the stress on families increases and there is less time or emotional space to care. Families, then, are characterized by significant differences among and within them, differences often not taken into account in providing public care.

Families are likely to be characterized by inequality among members and by a sexual division of labour that leaves women doing most of the domestic work. Women without paid work are dependent on the economic earnings of others or on the state, with all the dependency relations that are entailed. Those with incomes seldom earn as much as men, given the gap between male and female earnings. Children, and increasingly young adults, are also economically dependent, leaving them with less status than those who bring in the bulk of the income. Some families are characterized by violence and abuse, most of which is directed against women and children. Few have the kind of skills necessary to use oxygen masks and catheters, change wound dressings or provide support to someone with cancer. Many do not have appropriate physical space for the kinds of care required. While the nature of the human relationship is one of interdependency, the interdependency in households often means the dependency is unequal in ways that create significant differences in security, autonomy and rights.

When care moves home it usually means care by women because of assumptions about who should care, the failure to provide alternative public care, and men's higher wages, which mean it makes sense for the women in the house to sacrifice their paid jobs or adjust them to the care work. Estimates indicate that such families have been providing between 80 and 90 percent of all care, even before current moves to send care home. With most mothers in the labour force, and even mothers of small children now expected to work rather than remain home on welfare, few women have much time for additional care. Part-time employment is often so irregular that it cannot easily be accommodated to extra care work, and so low paid it may not be an alternative for many. The minority of women who have partners with full-time, relatively permanent and well-paid employment may also find it impossible to absorb this new care work, whether or not they want to provide it or think they should provide it, given the care responsibilities they already carry. The result may well be "compulsory altruism" for these women (Land and Rose 1985) while other women may simply not be able to provide the care sent to the community or to support a caring community. The additional pressure on families can disrupt or even sunder those that do fit the rosy picture of family life.

In other words, sending care to the community may mean undermining those communities and does not necessarily mean more local participation or control. As Stacey Oliker says on the basis of her research on welfare, "[W]e might find damage to personal networks and personal relationships, which could threaten families' capacities to care. The damage might take the form of constriction and greater fragility in networks, the replacement of caregiving support with support for subsistence, and a decline in communal commitments to care" (Oliker 2000:178). This does not leave much space for even more care. Without time, space, economic resources and other supports, all communities may be at similar risk, and innovation as well as participation, stifled.

LINKING PRIVATE AND PUBLIC SPHERES

Rapid state and economic expansion were not the only significant features of the welfare state. The "Golden Years" were also characterized by the development of clearer boundaries between the private and public spheres.

Within the formal economy, large fields of activity – including both those working directly for the government in the bureaucracy as "public servants" and those working indirectly in health, social services and education – came to be part of the broader public sector. Funding for these industries came primarily from governments, which highly regulated them through detailed legislation and reporting rules. Governments carried out their commitments to human rights and welfare mainly through them – pay and employment equity legislation, for example, applied primarily to the broader public sector. In Canada, almost all of the organizations in health, education, welfare and social services were nonprofit. Their services, in other words, were not produced for exchange in the market; they were not commodified. Those working in these industries were paid a wage, and thus their labour was commodified, but the services themselves were not. There was a specific logic at work for these employees and employers, with public service defined and treated differently from other market work. It is easier to focus on care when profits and payments are not required. Unions flourished, in part because there was one main funder and in part because governments had made commitments inside and outside the country regarding the kinds of rights that unions demanded.

At the same time as the distinction between the public and private sectors in the market became clearer, so did the distinction between the formal economy and the household. Feminists talked increasingly about the separation of public and private spheres. Many more women worked for pay in the market, outside the home. Many services previously associated with households became available for purchase in the market. Frozen foods and McDonald's hamburgers, machine-knit sweaters and residential care for the disabled all signalled this development. Although often described as moving women's work out of the home, much of the caring work provided in the market either by the state or the for-profit sector was quite different from the work that women had traditionally done in the home. More elderly, severely ill and disabled people are surviving, primarily as a result of public supports and access to highly technical medical care. The kind of care required by these people was never provided by women at home in the past, and the equipment and skills involved were most easily provided in institutional settings by people trained for the job. Medicalization drew further boundaries, identifying whole areas of not only bodies but also lives as appropriately treated by medical experts.

During this period, governments defined households as private domains, further supporting the separation. Prime Minister Trudeau talked about keeping the state out of the bedrooms of the nation. Divorce and abortion became easier, homosexuality and birth control were decriminalized, "spouse in the house" rules that involved state-supported inspection were relaxed. Households operated on the basis of a different logic, one based on relationships of blood, love and dependency rather than pay, although, as many feminists pointed out, their very privacy also meant they often hid hate, violence, poverty, inequality and various forms of abuse.

There were, then, some advantages to this sharpening division. Work in the public and private sectors was understood to be based on different motives. Some of women's skills were more likely to be recognized and paid for. It became easier to distinguish work from non-work time, and to resist extra loads as well as to fight for protections in each sphere. There were also, however, disadvantages. Boundaries often meant a greater focus on tasks, as jobs were broken down into clearly distinguishable and measurable parts. Medical intervention increased, often in inappropriate ways, with medical experts dominating care. Paid care was also defined as superior and, in efforts to increase the emphasis on this work as professional, more of the care was defined out of the work.

The separation was always far from complete. Many publicly funded services continued to be delivered by independent organizations rather than directly by government, and some at least operated like for-profit ones. Some services associated with the home, like child care, never became widely available. Indeed, welfare legislation was built on the assumption that women should stay home to care for young children. Few human services ever become mainly the responsibility of the state and many of the components in women's work remained the same, regardless of their location. Perhaps most importantly, as many feminists went on to make clear, households and private and public sector workplaces were never separate in the sense of operating independently of each other. The segregation of women's work in the labour force reflected and reinforced women's work in the household, and the reverse was also the case. Welfare states only ever took over some of the caring, leaving women to provide the rest. And some women continued to do home-work, taking paid employment within the home, while others took on only part-time or casual labour force work, as a means of juggling their two linked workplaces. Others, unable to find permanent full-time employment or child care, had little choice about taking on domestic work. As Gillian Pascal puts it, "a large part of state social policy consists in taking a small part of caring work into the public sphere" (Pascal 1997:75). Making only a small part of the care a public responsibility serves to perpetuate care as women's work, rendering much of the skill and labour invisible, and certainly making it undervalued. Indeed, states play a central role in what is done in private and public sectors in both senses of the terms, in determining what the boundaries are and in determining whether there are boundaries.

Restructuring the welfare state has brought about a further blurring of these separations. Within the public sector, the adoption of for-profit strategies and the contracting out of services makes the logic of market relationships central to these concerns. Partnerships between public and for-profit companies have similar consequences. The cutbacks to services mean either that more care has to be purchased in the market or that more of it must be undertaken by unpaid providers, either at home or in institutions. Both of these consequences of cutbacks further reduce the separation between private and public, contributing to the way public processes reinforce and penetrate private household ones.

Women who are paid carers find themselves teaching women in minutes how to do what took them years of training to learn, making it more difficult to distinguish both the work and the workers. At the same time, part-time, part-year, casual and self-employment are growing, supported by new technologies such as e-mail, cell phones and computer programs that make it possible to do paid work anywhere and to further mix paid and unpaid labour. These processes reflect, to some extent, women's increasing caring work, but they also serve to create women as carers in the private domain.

There is also some blurring along gender lines, with more men caring for their female or male partners as public care declines and fewer family members are available to care. These men are, however, more likely than their female counterparts to get help in their caring work from the state or from unpaid providers.

With more paid work now done at home, it is more difficult to separate the logics of households and market work or the skills required in each. With more paid and unpaid care provided in the home, the state moves more into the bedrooms of the nation. The conflicts among households, states and markets may be played out in these very rooms, among the women delivering care. Yet much abuse still remains hidden in the household and indeed may even be growing as those with high care needs are added to what may be a volatile mix.

The restructuring of work in the for-profit sector has also blurred many of the old separations. More men have moved into traditional women's jobs as work in the factories and the fields, producing things or extracting resources, has rapidly disappeared. More men have also taken on casual, part-time and short-term employment and many men's wages have stagnated or declined. Women, too, have made some shifts, with more of them doing traditional male work. As a result, men's employment patterns have become more similar to those of women. Within workplaces, some hierarchies have been flattened to blur the lines of authority and the boundaries between union and non-union areas. Multi-tasking breaks down old barriers among jobs and so "generic workers" – expected to do anything – become more common. Employers are also extending work hours and, in the extreme case of Ontario, the province has altered employment standards to allow for a sixty-hour week without overtime pay. Technologies make it possible to take more work home or to find workers more easily at home, making the distinction between home and work as difficult now for men to make, as it has long been for women.

With market logics more dominant and pervasive, so are differences related to economic resources. As more care work is done for low pay in the for-profit sector or for no pay at home, care work is less valued and more women have to combine it with other forms of low-paid work. But this collapsing does not happen for all women, given that it is still possible to substitute paid services for much of women's work. The more money a woman has, the better able she may be to maintain the separation among household, community, state and market; the better able she may be to maintain boundaries.

There are, however, some contrary trends. The most obvious is the greater emphasis within the public sector on carefully defined boundaries for what qualifies as care under public services. In health care for example, only the most acute, short-term interventions are now defined as necessary hospital care. The other aspects of care, those once combined in and provided by public sector institutions, are now defined outside the boundaries of high-tech care and thus as both less necessary, less skilled and less valuable, at least in an economic sense. Less obvious perhaps are the more rigid definitions of who qualifies for supports from the public sector. With the emphasis on individual responsibility, it is increasingly difficult to meet the criteria that separate the deserving from the undeserving. Consequently, more and more poor, old, immigrant, Aboriginal or sick women are defined as abusers of public care, and many of the boundaries between male and female jobs get reinforced by the increasing reliance on unpaid caregivers combined with continuing labour market segregation.

In sum, the components in the care work women do for pay in the public sector and in the private sector, and without pay in community organizations and households, are quite similar. It may be that the personal, hidden and unpaid nature of this work in households contributes to its low value in the labour force but it may also be that the low wages paid for women's work in the labour force contributes to the low value of their caring work in the home and the assignment of this work to women. Government and employer practices influence the distributions of power and of work and resources between women and men, as well as among women, and the extent to which women must or can care. They also powerfully influence the boundaries among spheres. In recent years, the impact of the new emphasis on markets in everything has blurred lines between the private and public in both senses of the terms; that is, between households and formal economies and between public and private sectors within the formal economy.

It is impossible to understand women's work and women's caring without examining the ways in which states, markets, communities and households penetrate and structure each other. The blurring of the lines among these sectors makes it more difficult to see the links and more difficult for women to draw boundaries, at the same time as more rigid lines are drawn in some areas in order to reduce public support.

PAYING FOR CARE

Care costs. Some of the costs are financial. Some are in time, in emotional and social resources, or in lost opportunities. These costs may be borne mainly by individuals, families, community organizations or governments. Sometimes all share in the costs, although they seldom do so in equal portions or in similar ways. Whatever the distribution, the ways in which costs are borne and shared have significant consequences for women. However, the issues go beyond what the costs are and who pays. They also include how payment is made and to whom, or through whom, it is made.

In Canada, the state provides most of the financial funding for paid care, but the payments take many forms. When the federal government decided to introduce public hospital care, it did so by funding services rather than individuals. These services are provided either directly by the government or, more commonly, by other nonprofit organizations paid to provide the care. With the exceptions of B.C. and Alberta that also require premiums, these services are funded entirely out of general government revenues and are provided without fees. The federal government set out the principles requiring that admission be determined by doctors and hospitals on the basis of medical necessity and that comprehensive care be universally available. Initially, most jurisdictions funded hospitals on the basis of demonstrated need but later switched to global funding systems. More recently, some have moved to paying on the basis of Diagnostic Related Groups, which link payment to the illnesses treated rather than providing overall budgets.

These systems of funding expanded access to hospital services dramatically and helped the many women employed in these public hospitals to make important gains in terms of wages and working conditions. Certainly, the location and nature of services provided did limit access for women in some areas of the country and did prevent some women from receiving appropriate care, but there can be little doubt that services provided without financial costs increase access for women. This payment system meant care was not linked to insurance provided through employment or direct private payments, especially important for women given their lower employer rates and pay levels. Women could choose among hospitals and had some choice about when to leave. Hospitals had every reason to admit any patients with health care needs and to provide them with as much care as they thought they required for as long as they thought necessary. Hospitals took the lion's share of health care spending and provided a wide range of services.

The principles of universality, accessibility and comprehensiveness remain but a combination of factors has led to some dramatic changes. Costs rose enormously, government coffers were seen to be empty, and there was a new set of values guiding state expenditures. Moreover, women's groups, among others, criticized the bureaucratic and authoritarian nature of institutions as well as the failure to respond to the needs of particular groups, at the same time as they argued that much care could be provided more appropriately elsewhere. Funding was cut and new techniques introduced. There was a new emphasis on both market approaches and a narrower definition of hospital care. Hospitals were managed more like for-profit concerns. Some hospitals were amalgamated and others closed or converted. Day surgery, outpatient services and shorter patient stays became the norm. While patients continued to be admitted, they required much more care and had less choice about how long to stay.

For the women paid to work there, this has meant they have to work harder under conditions that make it more difficult for them to do their work, to feel secure or to derive satisfaction from the work. It means they must rely more on relatives, especially female ones, and must cope with more frustrations. They have less time to teach, learn or care. They also have less autonomy and less control over what they do and how they do it as care procedures are increasingly standardized and monitored. With the highest recorded injury rates of any industry, they are clearly endangering their own health – and the strains of their work undoubtedly spill over into their households and communities, just as the work no longer done in hospitals does. For the women seeking care, less is provided in the fee-less sector while restructuring often means that the available care is much farther from home, making it not only more difficult for patients to access but also more difficult for friends or family to provide support.

The state also paid directly for medically necessary services provided and defined by doctors, but in this case usually on the basis of each service rather than on the basis of salaries or global budgets. Patients could not be charged fees here either and they had the right to choose the services of any doctor. This method of payment increased access and meant that many of the poorest and sickest could now get care. It also meant doctors could base their judgement more on care needs than costs. At the same time, however, it encouraged an emphasis on medical intervention and discouraged a focus on prevention, health promotion and care. That work was still left primarily to households and public health units. Although some physician services have been identified as no longer covered by public coffers and some limits put on fees, in general these have served to increase the emphasis on medical interventions, as have new approaches in hospitals. Meanwhile, public health, the other health service funded directly by the state and provided without fees, has been significantly reduced. This service not only helps keep people healthy, thus reducing care needs, it also helps women look after themselves and others in the home.

State funding for long-term care and home care, as well as other community services, is much more diverse. Most programs have strict eligibility criteria and require fees – and rising fees have been combined with stricter criteria. The more fees and eligibility criteria play a role, the more difficult it is to ensure equal access and the more care is left to the household. The same is true of day care services which, for the most part, are based on subsidies for the deserving poor rather than on funded centres open to all. As a result, there are growing gaps among those who receive and provide care. Moreover, more of the long-term, home and day care paid for from the public purse is provided by for-profit firms. For-profit firms necessarily spend some of their money on profits rather than care, putting considerable pressure on the women who work in these organizations to work harder and for less money than in the hospital sector.

Governments also fund individuals directly or indirectly, allowing them to purchase or provide care. Tax deductions to cover the costs of providing or receiving care can provide some support, but they do little to help those with low incomes. Means-tested allowances to purchase or provide care services are another option. In addition to offering resources, these allowances may give care recipients more choices about what kinds of care they receive and who provides it. They may also mean some pay for women who previously received no pay for providing care. Care allowances can thus mean some power shift. And they may be the only option in areas without other services. Such allowances raise a number of critical issues, however. The allowances are usually quite low, reinforcing the low value attached to women's work while confirming it as women's work. The personal arrangements may be exploitative for either the provider or the recipient, especially if there are no other options. Finally, with the care hidden in the household, it is difficult to assess its nature and quality.

Insurance companies also fund care, and are doing so increasingly as less care is provided through public services. Insurance companies have eligibility criteria both for joining insurance schemes and for what care and how much will be covered. They also require premiums, most of which are made available through workplace plans. Women are less likely than men to be covered at work but are more likely than men to be covered as spouses. They are less likely to be able to pay the premiums and, given that they live longer and use more services, it seems likely that they would more often be denied coverage. Women who have no employed partners, or who are poor, are thus left to rely on friends, families and charities, rather than insurance, for care. As services are delisted and public care made less accessible, more people rely on insurance, thus increasing differences in the right to care.

Charitable and religious organizations rely on both governments and gift-giving for their funds. Both sources are frequently variable and unreliable, making it difficult to provide either stable care or stable employment. Tax deductions are intended to encourage support for these organizations, but they mean that those with money make decisions at government expense about what care is provided. They may also be able to use their financial power to influence the criteria used for care.

Finally, individuals and families pay for care. As less care is provided in the public system and by insurance companies, more care must either be paid for out of private purses or be provided without pay. Those with economic resources will be able to buy care directly. And some women do fall into this category. However, most women have to find other means of getting or giving care. For those with few resources, this can mean they have and give no care at all. Even when paid care is provided, there are additional direct economic costs in providing care, costs such as drugs, bandages, and equipment. Equally important, women pay in terms of their paid employment and their own health; in terms of opportunities forgone and control over their lives. Families may be disrupted or even sundered, especially with the increasingly universal assumption that all families can care. Women are more likely than men to be left alone to care.

In sum, funding is about more than money. It also is about how, and with what criteria, funding is provided. Each method of funding has an impact on access to care and on the nature of care.

THINKING THROUGH SPACE

Not only social locations related to gender, class, race, culture and age matter. Physical location also plays a role in the nature of care provided and in the conditions for care.

In the move to shift care from institutions to communities, institutions have been portrayed as impersonal, bureaucratic, hierarchical, distant, expensive, lacking in privacy and even dangerous. By contrast, communities are characterized as personal, immediate, responsive to individual needs, cheaper, safer, private and more individual.

Yet institutions also mean more people, more equipment, more safety measures, more formal education and more opportunities for promotion. They also provide better pay and benefits to providers than communities do. Within institutions, people can work in teams that bring together a range of skills and provide mutual support. Such teams can also make both providers and care recipients feel safer and act more safely. They provide a place where you can go for help; a stable address for care. Moreover, institutions can provide some boundaries for providers and recipients, boundaries that help increase control and reduce some of the negative aspects of dependency. Equally important, public institutions funded on the basis of universal access can reduce gaps in access among recipients and help create decent working conditions for providers, while paid provision offers an important alternative or complement to unpaid care.

Communities, on the other hand, can mean isolation for providers and care recipients, isolation from both others with appropriate knowledge and who can offer social support or protection. Communities can also be dangerous, with privacy hiding violence, ignorance or lack of the means to provide adequate care. Equipment and facilities are less likely to be designed for specialized care and the crowding of care into inadequate space can have emotional costs for the whole community. Furthermore, community providers tend to be low-paid or unpaid and seldom have any benefits. Indeed, community care is cheaper primarily because the full range of costs is not counted and because the care may well be inferior to that provided in institutional settings. Perhaps most importantly, the gaps in care are much wider within communities both because it is less monitored or visible and because there are great inequalities among communities in terms of their resources. Communities remove the boundaries, creating more personal connections while increasing dependency and reducing control. Moreover, the move to communities assumes people have communities that can and will serve their care needs. As people move more within the country and around the globe, their communities of support often disappear.

Households are also often ill-equipped to provide care. In addition to the more obvious problems of having wheelchair access or room for a lift, the physical space may be unable to accommodate the demands for care without invading the space necessary for families to live, enormously escalating the tensions of daily interactions. Families vary significantly in their capacity to make such accommodations. And, of course, some families have no home at all.

The point is not to reverse the claims, arguing that institutions are better than communities. Rather, the point is to raise questions about the move out of institutions and suggest this be re-examined, taking a different perspective. Instead of setting these up as good/bad alternatives, we should be asking how we can make both better, injecting what is good about each into the other and thinking about the impacts on both providers and recipients. And when we are redesigning these spaces, we should also be thinking about how their internal physical structures promote or impede care.

The Location of Care

Combined with a shift from institutions into communities is the development of giant institutions and the elimination of smaller ones. Justified as more efficient and effective, these massive structures are clearly important in providing high-tech, skilled care. However, they also move care further from home, making it difficult for care recipients to connect with their communities just as they need the support most. Indeed, all the issues raised about bad institutions can apply to them. Despite evidence to support a claim that some highly specialized care facilities are necessary, there is less evidence to support the claim that most care institutions should take this form or that giant organizations are necessarily less expensive in the long term.

In a country the size of Canada, space is obviously about more than the size of institutions. Canada is a highly urbanized country, with many of our cities divided internally by race, culture and class. Where care is located within the cities and the extent to which the cities respond to the particular needs of their different populations are clearly questions that need to be addressed in thinking about care. Location can determine access not only in terms of the physical distance required to travel and the cost or availability of transportation but also in terms of the cultural space between providers and care recipients. With sufficient populations that can demand and sustain them, cities may well be better placed to provide for a variety of needs. It is possible, for example, to offer respite services that can accommodate several languages, to build long-term care facilities that serve Catholics, and to create community centres and programs that cater specifically to Black teens.

Urban dwellers are often better placed than their rural counterparts. As geographers Greg Halseth and Allison Williams explain, the "general problem of service provision in small, geographically isolated, rural communities is exacerbated by government policy that fails to recognize the unique circumstances of these non-urban places" (Halseth and Williams 1999:29). Although rural areas, like other communities, are often portrayed as caring and sharing, there may be few people around to care and share as young people leave home in search of work, shopping moves to the city and fewer people are required to work the farm or the boat. Even women with economic resources may find it impossible to find paid providers to locate in these regions and unpaid providers may find themselves working alone without a safety net. Those who are a minority within Canadian society are likely to be a very small minority in rural areas, leaving them with little choice about support for care that addresses their particular needs. Yet it is possible, as Halseth and Williams demonstrate using the example of rural Ontario, that with state support communities can build integrated public services that support "community wellness" for unpaid providers (Halseth and Williams 1999).

Canadian-born residents may also be better placed than the foreign-born, because space may separate the latter not only from people who can provide care but also from the culturally familiar. Even for the Canadian-born, however, frequent moves to follow education and jobs or, especially in the case of the retired, to seek cheaper housing, may separate both relatives and cultures. Lack of public transport can also make care problematic, especially for women, who are more likely than men to rely on it. Moreover, more and more women have to travel extensively for their work, moving them far from their care work.

Questions of space may also be viewed from the perspectives of the different people involved in care. For the day care employee, the centre is a workspace; for the child, a play space; and for the mother a space which may be either supportive of her or undermining to her, or perhaps both at the same time. Similarly, a long-term care facility is a home for residents, a workplace for paid providers and sometimes a space to be avoided by relatives who feel guilty about placing their mothers there. For families, home may be a place for entertaining friends; for the care recipients a place where they need quiet comfort; and for the paid care providers a workplace that should be ordered in a manner that meets their standards of care. Thus, each of the participants may have different, and conflicting, space needs – the care provider may want a smoke-free workplace that has accessible equipment to help with lifts, while the care recipient wants to smoke in what is now home and may not want this home to be crowded with equipment that is a reminder of frailty.

Space is thus also about social relations. It can make better care possible or it can undermine care. It can promote or mitigate against conflict. It can support or undermine unpaid providers or do both at the same time. There can be space for a hug, an often unmeasured but critical component of care for provider and recipient; or a hug may be ruled out by the structural arrangements.

In short, space matters. Location also has an impact on the work of unpaid providers delivering people to care and seeking support in their caring. So does the kind of physical space in which care is provided. Although this section raises only some of the issues related to space and care, they should be sufficient to show that physical location must be taken into account in understanding care.

THINKING ABOUT TIME

Space issues are linked to time issues. Care is required and provided in different time frames, as well as in different locations and the two may be related. So, for example, if hospitals are now concentrated in one urban centre, the time it takes for unpaid providers to get to their unpaid work will be lengthened. Indeed, the time it takes may make it impossible to provide this unpaid care. There may be space for a hug, but no time. And like space, time can be viewed from number of different perspectives.

Perhaps the most obvious time issue is the difference between the short term and the long term. An emphasis on markets and costs encourages an emphasis on short-term financial expenditures. However, what is cheaper in the short term may be more expensive over the long term. The short-term view can mean increasing the workloads of paid and unpaid providers now in order to cut costs. But the long-term costs for the women who provide care may include deteriorating health, lost job opportunities, disrupted communities and poverty in old age. At the same time, it may mean deteriorating health for those who receive care. It is now fashionable in policy circles to stress the importance of the early years for later life – that is, to take a longer view – but children are too often examined as if they had no care providers who themselves have needs that must be addressed in order to offer good care. Care providers too grow old, and their needs in old age are influenced by the care they provide now and how they must provide that care.

The focus on the short term also obliterates the way people move through periods of dependency and providing throughout the life cycle. We are all dependent as children, but in turn the majority of us care for dependent children. The teenagers who suffer today from depression may as adults support young people with similar concerns. Those who need considerable help after major surgery this week may next month provide care for a friend in similar circumstances. The same elderly who are named today as the threat to our health care system were yesterday providing care and may still be doing so today in some form. People with lifelong disabilities often also have periods in which they too can provide support, or they may provide this support in different ways.

Time is also about time of life. The needs and resources of women who arrive in Canada in their sixties are different from those of women who come as infants. The time for caring that a young woman beginning a career has is quite different from the time a retired woman has. The time a woman with young children and a job has is not the same as the time the mother without paid work and children at home has. However, in none of these cases can we simply assume any of the women has time to care.

The lumping of care into a single category may hide the significant differences in the time required for care. People who have day surgery usually require intense support for a limited period of time. Some people with disabilities require limited care each day for life; some require intense care for life. And their life expectancy may be short or long. Children require not only different amounts of time as they age but also different kinds of time. The same is true of people with different illnesses. Care may take the same amount of time each day or a variable amount of time each day. It may be daily or occasional. It may be limited now but increase with each day. This care time is also related to space. It may be more possible to account for the needs of someone who is severely ill for a finite period of time within a confined household but much more difficult to do so if long-term care is required. These time dimensions obviously have significantly different consequences for providers. Women are more likely than men to do the care that is done every day and over long periods of time.

The time it takes to care may have clear boundaries and be spatially confined. This is more likely to be the case for paid providers and for men than it is for women, and especially for those who provide unpaid care. Such boundaries are more difficult to draw when provider and recipient share the same space, when care needs are chronic, or when a single person is the primary care provider. The lack of time boundaries can make independence and separation difficult or impossible. Providers can find themselves in situations in which they have no time for themselves, no time away from caring.

Waiting times are a further issue. How long care recipients wait for an appointment or wait in line after the appointment is made has an impact not only on their time but also on the time of the care provider. Some of this time is obvious as mother and daughter sit together in the emergency room. But the anxiety, as well as other health consequences, of such waits can also mean more time is required for the rest of care. Limits on care time also have obvious consequences for unpaid care. Within and outside institutions, women often find themselves making up for the care not provided because paid care time has been cut to a minimum, and often based on the assumption that unpaid providers will fill in the rest of the time. At home, care is often required twenty-four hours a day but public care seldom provides for more than a few hours. Similarly, respite time is often so short it simply leaves time for frantically completing other unpaid work rather than enjoying some respite.

Like space, time may appear differently to each of the participants. For the employer, time is money and therefore every effort is made to reduce care to the most obviously necessary and easily measured tasks. This involves controlling as precisely as possible the time each person takes to provide care. For the employee, control may be as important as income, and control includes the capacity to decide how long to spend with each care recipient as well as on each task. For the care recipient, control over the time spent is equally important. This may mean getting care provided as quickly as possible or taking as long as possible, but in either case it requires some control over time. What is a long time for the provider may be a short time for the recipient. As with space, resources can help caregivers gain more control over their time. However, this is not necessarily the case – the woman executive, for example, may have no time to care, even though she has the money to buy time from someone else to provide care.

Those advocating for unpaid caregivers have frequently argued for time budget studies, and have successfully argued for Census counting of care time. The purpose is to make the care visible so it can be valued and supported, financially or otherwise. Although the purpose is laudable, the solution of counting care time is problematic. Care time is difficult to count in part because it is hard to define and the boundaries are so unclear. This is especially the case when it overlaps in households with other kinds of work, paid or unpaid. Moreover, those who provide care often do not define it as care time – is baking cookies that will be eaten by a family with a disabled child leisure, domestic work or care work? And how long do cookies take? Does sitting down for a cup of tea with a neighbour dying of cancer count as care and how long does tea take? Similarly, women who have been looking after their spouses all their lives may not count the laundry and cooking they do for their frail and dependent spouses as care time. In the effort to make care visible, the pressure on counting tasks and reducing care to such tasks may increase at the same time as the total time involved is underestimated. This underestimation, in turn, may serve as an excuse to send more care work home to be done by those whose time pressures are rendered invisible by these counting techniques.

In sum, time interacts with space and both matter. Time, too, is about social relations. Time is a critical aspect of care, one that needs to be considered in order to understand the demands on providers and the alternatives available to them.

EMPOWERMENT

Empowerment is, like globalization, a term covering many notions of how people gain and keep power.

In policy circles, it is often talked about as increasing choice. And choice, in turn, is intended to mean consumer choice, or the right to buy. This is the kind of choice that is meant by the introduction of non-public health care services, services that could be purchased instead of using public ones. It is the kind of empowerment meant by a voucher system for purchasing child care or home care. There are, however, two basic problems with this kind of choice, in addition to those described earlier as problems with markets in general in relation to public goods and services. First, when everyone uses the same public system they have an interest in ensuring that the public system is good. As soon as they can buy alternative care directly, they have less interest in maintaining a public system and indeed may object to supporting it. The result is poor care for the poor unable to afford the private system, most of whom are women. Second, consumer choices are usually individual rather than collective, and those with more consumer power have more choice. This too means greater inequality, and even less choice for the many women without this kind of power. Consumer choice in care thus simply means more power for those who already have it and more work and less care for those who do not.

Empowerment is also often used to mean accountability, a concept that itself has several meanings. Increasingly, accountability in care means counting. In the name of accountability, ensuring quality and evidence-based decision-making, more and more data are being produced by care organizations. With all the new technology, we count the number of beds used and how frequently, the number of services provided and how often, the number of caesarean sections performed per surgeon and where they are done, the number of children taught by each teacher for how long, the number of tasks performed per provider in how many minutes, to name only some of the numbers collected in this rush to accountability. Although such numbers are often useful in decision-making, much depends not only on what is counted and how it is counted, but also about what is done with those numbers. If they are used to justify decision-making by experts in ways that exclude women, then they can mean disempowerment rather than empowerment. Furthermore, arguments for accountability defined as accounting in particular ways may put considerable burdens on communities that must produce such accounts in order to be eligible for support in providing care.

Regionalization and deinstitutionalization have also been characterized as forms of empowerment. Sending care and responsibility closer to home has been presented as a means of responding to local needs. Regionalization may mean more women are involved in decision-making in local boards, especially if they are elected. However, much depends on the resources and power given to these regional boards. If they are more about responsibility for cuts and decisions about creating services, then regionalization may be disempowering. Furthermore, local decision-making, especially under conditions of severe restraint, may mean that the needs of particular groups such as lesbians and immigrant women are ignored. Sending care closer to home could mean care recipients have more choices about how their lives are structured, but, under current conditions and without public service support, it simply means more work for women and less control over their lives when they provide care. One woman who has looked after two very ill, elderly parents for years recently wrote to us to say she was "under house arrest." Clearly, care closer to home has not meant empowerment for her.

For paid caregivers, power involves the right to make daily decisions about what should be done for and with a patient. It also involves a say over when, if, where and how they work. Restructuring has created considerable disruption for these workers, reducing in the process their sense of security and control. Simultaneously, in the name of increasing efficiency new managerial strategies have been developed precisely to reduce the control these providers have over their work. Although Total Quality Management and other such schemes have been introduced in the name of increasing participation, there is little evidence that they have actually empowered workers and some evidence to indicate that the schemes reduce the power of their unions. For unpaid providers, restructuring has also disrupted familiar service structures. This alone would not be a problem. Indeed, it may even be an advantage if it led to the promised "one-stop shopping" that provided access to a full range of coordinated services and those helping others to get care could save time and steps. However, when combined with cutbacks on care and limits to care, it may simply mean that there is coordinated denial and that providers feel they have less say over what care is available to assist them in their care work. With paid workers entering households both to assess the need for care and to provide it, unpaid providers may feel disempowered by rules set elsewhere and applied within their own homes by professionals who seem to have power.

The relationship between care provider and care receiver is also about power. How power is balanced depends to some extent on the alternatives available to each, as well as on their resources. Care receivers may be disempowered by their dependency, a dependency that increases as access to public alternatives decreases.

Empowerment is about gaining access to resources. Some of these resources are material, like income and services, or drugs and diapers. Some are political, like the right to participate fully in decision-making in ways that have an impact, or the right to equal pay and other employment protections, or the right to education and information. Some are social, like having time and space for friends and relaxation. Some are symbolic, like having care recognized as work that requires time, space, time, money, physical capacity, emotional involvement and social support. The more resources distributed by market mechanisms, the greater the disparities in resources and thus in power.

WHAT IS IT ABOUT CARE?

Care is a complex concept. It necessarily involves a relationship, whether the care is provided by paid or unpaid strangers, friends or family. It involves a relationship because it is people who need care, people who must communicate, respond, relate. It is thus a reciprocal rather than one-way process. It is a relationship that often involves intimacy and may involve dealing with our most intimate or personal needs, even our very definitions of self. And because this is a human relationship, it also involves emotions. The emotions may be strong or relatively weak, sometimes one and then the other, or both at the same time. They may involve love or hate and often both these contradictory emotions simultaneously. They may be mainly about concern for another human being who has needs that may well be ours someday. They may be about how others perceive our needs.

The care relationship brings together individuals with specific histories, specific locations, specific needs. It involves whole, complicated people embedded in networks of social relationships. And this is as true of the care providers as it is of the care recipients. While there are clearly general patterns of needs and there are clearly ways we can develop general strategies for addressing them, each relationship requires a sensitivity to the particular persons involved. So, for example, it is necessary to develop procedures for treating Alzheimer's, but how those with Alzheimer's are treated depends on their circumstances and conditions. Someone who has survived the Holocaust may have a particular aversion to any form of restraint while someone who was born in Japan may need particular kinds of food in order to feel safe. What is vital is specialness, rather than sameness, at the level of care in the individual case. Rules need to be interpreted in the context of the specific; equity needs to be defined in the context of understanding difference.

Care relationships are thus diffuse rather than clearly defined. The boundaries for care are usually difficult to draw in terms of what is done, how long it is done and where it is done. Care work is about much more than a series of tasks precisely because it involves verbal and non-verbal communications and emotions that are difficult to make visible and measure, specify on paper and assign as discrete items. Certainly we can tease out tasks that are part of care and we can determine skills required for the work. Indeed, recognizing the skill involved in caring is essential if we are to ensure that care is not only made visible and valued but also safely delivered. Recognizing the skilled nature of the work is also necessary if we are to ensure that we do not assume that all women can and should provide all care. We can also outline needs in quite detailed ways. But the process that transforms procedures into care is much more blurred, more difficult to express. So are the boundaries on needs. Certainly we need to have some boundaries, otherwise care work will be endless and especially burdensome. We need as well to draw some lines to make sure that caring *about* someone does not mean you must care *for* them. We have to realize, however, that precisely because care is about people's needs the boundaries cannot easily be precisely determined according to standardized rules and procedures that fail to allow considerable individual judgement and control.

The character of care relationships varies with individuals, locations, external pressures and training. Notions of professional distance created by training and pay shape the emotional involvement, but if distance means complete detachment it is difficult to think of it as care. Skills need to be acquired, often certified and certainly practiced, but some of them are acquired through experience and early in life, in ways that are difficult to recognize or assess through formal educational means. Those who are paid and highly educated are more likely to have authority than are those who are not, and they are also more likely to share the care with others than are unpaid caregivers. For unpaid care providers, the responsibility may be defined as the result of a relationship, while for paid ones responsibility may be defined in terms of professional oaths and ethics. Nevertheless, both paid and unpaid providers feel responsible for the people who need care. What we need are strategies to ensure that it is possible to fulfill these different responsibilities without creating more inequalities among women and without locking in or reinforcing poor care.

The nature of care contrasts sharply with the notions, practices and pressures in most labour market work. In the market, efforts are made to define work in terms of tasks, to have clear boundaries in time and space, to promote distance, to develop standardized procedures and to define equity as sameness. Responsibility is achieved more through hierarchy, pay and bureaucratic control than through relationships or guilt. Like the boundaries between private and public, however, the boundaries between care work and other forms of work are becoming even more blurred.

Deborah Stone argues that we need "to make the essence of caring visible, not so much in order to make it countable and rewardable, but rather, in order to render clear what it is that we want to provide in the public sphere" (Stone 2000:91). It is, in other words, important to recognize what is valuable and critical to keep the care in care, wherever it is done. But, we would add, it is necessary to do the same in the private sphere as well. While precise boundaries and standard procedures limit the possibilities for choices and care through paid work, lack of boundaries and procedures may limit choices and care through unpaid work. Similarly, recognizing the whole person, their special needs, their personal histories and the emotional aspects of care is critical, but placing too much emphasis on both may make caring impossible in either sphere, by paid or unpaid providers. There are dangers in the stress on relationships because this stress can be used to make paid workers contribute far more than the hours for which they are paid and unpaid ones work far beyond the point of exhaustion. The failure to recognize relationships may make care work like factory work, limiting possibilities for both providers and recipients.

Without both supports and alternatives, care for paid and unpaid care workers can become a burden without end. Without collective responsibility for care, those with the least resources are those most likely to have the greatest burden at the same time as they will find it difficult to provide care. By making care visible and beginning by making it the objective, we can then work towards solutions that give as many people as possible the right to care. Care is the objective, not the problem.

GUIDELINES FOR THINKING ABOUT CARE

1. *Both lumping and slicing are required.* It necessary to understand not only what women share and how they differ, but also to take different approaches to the same issues and situations. It is equally necessary to resist definitions of women as "natural" caregivers, exposing the social relations, processes and structural arrangements that create women as primary carers and do so in different ways for different women.
2. *Contexts matter.* Contexts are most notably provided by global tendencies and realities, states, markets, communities and families. Contexts also include notions about these, as well as about women, race, culture, sexuality, equity and age. All play a role in shaping women's caring, although the role they play is contradictory. It is important to recognize that these contexts are created by human hands, including those of women. There are thus choices to be made and women participate in these decisions, albeit often in unequal ways.
3. *It is important to assess boundaries and overlaps, linking public and private spheres.* Recent developments have served to blur boundaries between private and public sectors of the economy and between formal economy and household. While private and public spheres in both senses of the terms have always influenced each other, the influence may well be stronger the more boundaries are blurred. In any case, it is necessary to explore not only how each influences the other but also how the structure of boundaries influences women's caring.
4. *Payment is critical.* What the costs involved in care are, who pays and how they pay are all questions that need to be addressed in understanding women's caring. The costs include much more than money, and the methods of payment much more than providing financing. As access to

resources becomes more critical in accessing care, differences among women increase.

5. *Time and space are factors in care.* Time and space are both resources and limitations, and are linked to each other and to differences among women.

6. *Empowerment must be defined in ways that understand that power is about access to resources.* The resources are material, political, social and symbolic, and profoundly influence whether women can participate in making decisions about their own lives.

7. *Care is the objective, not the problem.* All human beings want and need care, although their needs and wants vary with for example age, location and ability.

The reason for developing our understanding of women's work in general and their caring work in particular is in order to allow this understanding to provide the basis for creating conditions that allow women the right to care in ways that take their needs and capacities into account.

An earlier version of this chapter was commissioned and published by the Maritime (now Atlantic) Centre of Excellence on Women's Health as a "concept paper" to inform The Healthy Balance Research Program, a community alliance for health research on women's unpaid caregiving. Further information on this program is available at <www.medicine.dal.ca/mcewh>. We appreciate the support provided us by the Program. Responsibility for the chapter's content rests of course with us alone.

References

Abel, Emily K. (2000). "A Historical Perspective on Care," pp. 8-14 in Madonna Harrington Meyer (ed.), *Care Work: Gender, Labour and the Welfare State.* London: Routledge.

Brandth, Berit and Elin Kvande. (2001). "Flexible Work and Flexible Fathers." Paper presented to the conference on "Rethinking Gender, Work and Organization," Keele University, UK, June 2001.

Cardozo, Andrew. (1996). "Lion Taming: Downsizing the Opponents of Downsizing," pp. 303-36 in Gene Swimmer (ed.) *How Ottawa Spends 1996-97: Life Under the Knife.* Ottawa: Carleton University Press, 1996).

Chang, Grace. (2000). *Disposable Domestics: Immigrant Women Workers in the Global Economy.* Cambridge, MA: South End Press.

Estes, Carroll L., Karen W. Linkins and Elizabeth A. Binney. (2001). "Critical Perspectives on Aging," pp. 23-44 in Carroll L. Estes and Associates, *Social Policy and Aging*. London: Sage.

Glucksmann, Miriam. (2000). *Cottons* Stacey J. *and Casuals: The Gendered Organization of Labour in Time and Space*. London: British Sociological Association.

Gough, Ian. *Global Capital, Human Needs and Social Policies*. New York: Palgrave, 2000.

Halseth, Greg and Allison Williams. (1999). "Guthrie House: A Rural Community Organizing for Wellness," pp. 29 in *Health and Place* 5(1):27-44.

Klein, Naomi. (2000). *No Logo: Taking Aim at the Brand Bullies*. Toronto: Knopf Canada, 2000.

Land, H. and H. Rose. (1985). "Compulsory Altruism for Some or an Altruistic Society for All?" in P. Bean, J. Ferris and D. Whynes (eds.), *In Defense of Welfare*. London: Tavistock.

National Forum on Health. (1997). *Canada Health Action: Building on the Legacy. Vol. II, Synthesis Reports and Issues Papers*, "The Need for an Aboriginal Health Institute in Canada." Ottawa: Minister of Public Works and Government Services.

Oliker, Stacey J. (2000). "Examining Care at Welfare's End," pp. 167-85 in Madonna Harrington Meyer (ed.), *Care Work: Gender, Labour and the Welfare State*. London: Routledge.

Pascal, Gillian. (1997). *Social Policy: A New Feminist Analysis*. London: Routledge.

Pierson, Christopher. (1999). *Beyond the Welfare State: The New Political Economy of Welfare,* Second Edition. Oxford: Blackwell.

Shields, John and B. Mitchell Evans. (1998). *Shrinking The State: Globalization and Public Administration "Reforms."* Halifax: Fernwood.

Stone, Deborah. (2000). "Caring by the Book," pp. 89-111 in Madonna Harrington Meyer (ed.), *Care Work: Gender, Labour and the Welfare State*. London: Routledge.

Ward, Kathryn (ed.). (1990). *Women Workers and Global Restructuring*. Ithaca, NY: Cornell University Press, 1990.

Whitfield, Dexter. (2001). *Public Service or Corporate Welfare: Rethinking the Nation State in the Global Economy*. London: Pluto Press.

Yalnizyan, Armine. (1998). "A Litmus Test for Democracy: The Impact of Ontario Welfare Changes on Single Mothers," *Studies in Political Economy* 66, Autumn 2001.

One Hundred Years of Caregiving

Pat Armstrong and Olga Kits

Caregiving is not a simple act but rather a complex social relationship – one embedded in personal histories and located within specific conditions. These relationships can be found throughout our society and in a multitude of forms. Caregiving exists within health care institutions and in hostels, in households and on the street. Where it happens, and with whom, changes over time and with place, even for the same individuals. Partners and friends, mothers and fathers, daughters and sons, relatives and strangers, old and young participate in caregiving, although there are clear patterns linked to gender, age and social circumstance. Informal caregiving is usually unpaid, done with little formal training and based on an existing relationship. Yet even the distinction between formal and informal care is far from simple. Some relatives are paid for such informal care; some begin as strangers; many have become quite skilled at caregiving and share the job with those who are part of the formal system.

To help sort through this complexity, this chapter begins with a discussion of the diversity in caregiving relationships. It then moves on to consider what changed and did not change significantly in these relationships throughout the twentieth century. On the basis of this exploration of history and diversity, the final sections set out a framework for assessing legislation, regulations and policy that influence caregiving among adults.

RECOGNIZING CAREGIVING IN ALL ITS DIVERSITY

What is Involved in Caregiving?

Caregiving among adults comes in an incredible variety of forms. The following stories, based on actual personal histories, convey only some of the variety in caregiving relationships, only some of the complexity and only some of the forms caregiving takes.

Marie and her partner, Louise, live with Louise's mother, Monique. Monique has severe bronchial problems that require considerable medical attention and treatments she cannot manage on her own. She cannot be left alone either. Working for the government and covered by a union contract, Marie does have the right to some care time and she would be happy to use it to stay with Monique, a woman whose company she thoroughly enjoys. It is not entirely clear, however, that this right extends to her partner's mother. Marie has already told her employer that she must leave at 5:00 pm each day so Louise can go to her job. This is her right under her contract, but she may well be jeopardizing her chances for promotion by doing so. She would very much like to be able to transfer some of her benefits to Louise, who has no such rights at her workplace and who has to work odd hours in order to accommodate her care work and meet her economic needs. As the primary caregivers, Marie and Louise recognize that they need a break from their double days and do this by ensuring that each year they take a two-week vacation away. Their incomes allow this, but do not extent to paid replacements. To go away means arranging with some seven friends and relatives to replace them while they are gone.

Himani and Wassem had twenty years of satisfying marriage before their son, Paresh, started acting in disturbing ways. In the three years it took for a diagnosis of schizophrenia, their marriage fell apart. Himani was left to care for their adult son alone and with little income. Many days with Paresh are fine, even fun. But now when Himani sees the signs she recognizes as indicating a bad period ahead, she often cannot get the help she needs from the formal system. For her, this means facing a sometimes violent episode without assistance.

Once a week, Katherine picks up her friend Laura and goes with her to the breast cancer support group. Laura's husband is away during the week, and in any case does not see what use he would be in such a place. Unlike Laura's professional colleagues, Katherine is an actress who has time during the day to spend with her friend. On the way into the clinic, Katherine often meets another actor taking someone to the HIV/AIDS clinic across the road. Organized by the gay community, the volunteers not only offer transport but also provide the kind of information necessary to access services and manage care.

Roberto had turned 84 the day he had to struggle up the stairs with his wife, Maria. Maria's surgery had failed to solve her medical problem and she had come home to die. Although frail himself, Roberto was determined to provide Maria with the kind of care she had so often provided for him. With most of his relatives back in Italy, he had to do as much as he could himself, especially with their sons so far away and caring for their own families. Home care helped, but not for many long hours in the day and Maria did not like the food they cooked. He still had to bath, feed, dress and toilet her when they were gone.

Sam and Marcia learned quite soon after their baby, Sarah, was born that she had severe disabilities that would undermine her development. Sarah requires total and specialized care, 24 hours a day. Both parents need their paid jobs in order to survive economically, especially with the extra costs created by their daughter's care needs. They manage because they found an excellent residential care facility that provides skilled and comforting care during the week. They visit Sarah regularly during the week and bring her home on weekends. However, the government is constantly threatening their funding so much of their time is taken up with pleading for public support. This precarious support is a constant strain, one that puts enormous stress on their relationship.

In addition to strictly medical care, the forms of care can be thought of as falling into four broad, overlapping categories. The most pervasive form is the management of care (Rosenthal and Martin-Matthews 1999). Almost all caregivers are involved in care management, but some caregivers are primarily managers. They find out about, and arrange for, formal services as well as ensuring that the formal services are received. They act like case managers, determining hours of service and eligibility, making appointments and convincing care recipients to participate. They mediate between care recipients and paid care providers, and advocate on behalf of recipients for care inside or outside the home. This organization of care not only involves negotiation among paid providers and with the care recipient it also involves negotiations among informal providers. Managing money, providing financial assistance, completing forms, assembling documents and organizing test results are all part of care management. Equally important, care management usually requires decision-making, often without the active participation of the person needing care. Each aspect of organizing care may involve conflicts: conflicts among formal and informal providers, conflicts between the groups and conflicts among any of the providers and the care recipient. This organization also requires cooperation among all of these participants and needs to be done even for people living in institutional settings. The need for such "orchestration of care," bureaucratic management and financial assistance (Rosenthal and Martin-Matthews 1999) varies over time, with illness and in relation to the availability of public support and services.

Another common form of caregiving involves what is known as Instrumental Activities of Daily Living (IADL). When people become ill, have day surgery, are released early from hospital, have more long-term disabilities or simply become frailer with old age, they require assistance with cooking, shopping, cleaning, laundry and home maintenance tasks. They may also need help getting around, within and outside the house. Residential care reduces the need for most, but not all, of this support. People may require assistance with only some of these tasks, or with all of them.

Some people require more than assistance understanding which services to use or with daily survival in their homes. They need direct help with much more personal and medical aspects of care. This third form of care is referred to as assistance with the Activities of Daily Living (ADL) and includes dressing, bathing, eating, using the toilet, brushing teeth and combing hair. It also includes taking medications, inserting needles and using a variety of equipment such as catheters, oxygen masks and feeding tubes. Here, too, residential care fills much of the need but still must be supplemented by informal caregivers in many cases.

Finally, there is the form of care that should pervade all the others but may also exist on its own. Everyone requires social and emotional support, but those who have undergone surgery, live with disabilities or live into frail old age have particular needs for companionship, for touch, for listeners and talkers and for comfort of all sorts, especially if they are not able to leave their home or institution. The need is particularly great in the case of palliative care. Caregivers may be engaged in only one of these forms, but many provide all four forms of care.

What Care is Provided?

What care is provided depends on a range, and mix, of factors. Government policies play a critical role in what care is provided, especially in terms of formal services. The *Canada Health Act 1984* requires that all medically necessary care provided by a doctor or hospital be offered to Canadian residents without charge and in an accessible manner. As care moves outside these boundaries, however, there is no national standard for formal, public care. This is why the National Forum on Health, a group appointed by Prime Minister Chrétien to advise on health policy, recommended national home care and pharmacare programs (National Forum on Health 1997). The Forum had little to say about long-term care facilities, although they too are largely outside the *Canada Health Act.*

Given that health care is primarily a provincial responsibility and that many of the services required in relation to informal caregiving are not included in the *Canada Health Act*, there are significant provincial variations in the supports available to informal caregivers and recipients. In terms of home care, while all provinces provide professional services such as nursing and physiotherapy without charge some charge user fees for home making, personal care, housecleaning or transportation. Some provide supplies and equipment without cost while others charge; some cover required medications while others do not. Some have extensive provisions for respite care while others provide very limited access. There is also considerable variation in eligibility rules and in the limits placed on services, creating even greater differences in supports available (Canadian Home Care Association 1998; Morris et al. 1999).

Ontario, for example, has established maximums of "80 hours of homemaking services per month for the first month; and 60 hours thereafter" and four nursing visits per day as maximums regardless of need (Canadian Home Care Association 1998:2) and has introduced user fees for drugs purchased under the public plans for the elderly, the disabled and those on welfare. By contrast, B.C.'s policy is to make community nursing "available 7 days a week, 24 hours a day" and home support services have a maximum of 120 hours per month, although more can be provided if a supervisor approves the additional hours (Canadian Home Care Association 1998:2). Moreover, B.C. has a universal pharmacare program and no or low user fees for particular groups (Bacovsky 1997). Access to institutional facilities also differs somewhat across provinces. While only 1 percent of Canadians live in such facilities (Trottier et al. 2000:49) the eligibility requirements, the location, the number of beds available, the nature of the services provided and the fees charged vary in ways that limit options for those caregivers and care recipients who need such services.

Government policies on direct and indirect financial support also influence the care provided. Direct financial support for care providers is quite limited and equally varied. Seven provinces and the Northwest Territories have "self-managed" care programs that provide either cash or service vouchers that allow care recipients to arrange their own care. The amounts are small and based on a means test. Most provincial financial support, however, comes indirectly through the tax system for deductions related to medical expenses, attendant allowances and disability. Since 1998, the federal Government has offered the Caregiver Tax Credit. This allows those who live with and care for an elderly relative to claim up to $400, if the claimant's annual income is less than $13,853 (Jenson and Jacobzone 2000). These deductions and credits mean little to the many low-income women who provide care, given that they have little actual income from which to deduct the taxes and that they may have "to absorb the cost of additional caregiving services before being eligible for reimbursements" (Keefe and Fancey 1997:256). There is, however, little research on the impact of direct financial compensation programs on caregivers or recipients (Keefe and Fancey 1997).

Access to formal services and other government financial supports for caregivers are clearly important to both care providers and care recipients. Yet, contrary to much popular discussion, the availability of formal care does not automatically mean that less informal care is provided. Indeed, study after study demonstrates that between 85 percent and 90 percent of care is provided informally (Ontario Ministry of Community and Social Services 1991; Denton 1997; Connidis 1983). Even these figures may understate the amount of informal care provided, given that "it is probably also the case that a lot more help is exchanged in families than is ever reported in surveys because people do not consciously think about what they are doing in providing help" (Rosenthal and Stone 1999:9). This is particularly the case for women who may see their caregiving work as a simple extension of usual practices. As a variety of researchers explain, for women, caring about someone is very often equated with caring for them and so the work and the skill of care become invisible in the process (Dalley 1988; Neysmith 2000; Finch and Groves 1983).

Informal and formal care are complementary rather than alternative forms of support (Rosenthal and Martin-Matthews; 1999; Chappell and Blandford 1991; Penning 2000; Keefe and Fancey 1997).

Instead of replacing informal caregivers, formal services are more likely to fill in when there are no informal caregivers or to provide some services that are supplemental to informal care (Denton 1997). As a study conducted for Statistics Canada concludes, "the informal network operates in concert with the formal delivery system" (Wilkins and Beaudet 2000:45) and the availability of formal services does not necessarily mean families and friends shirk their responsibilities. Nor does access to formal services mean people rush to use them. The overwhelming majority of health problems are managed through self-care. And "most people who consult a physician have tried treating themselves before seeking medical advice" (Morrongiello and Gottlieb 2000:38-39). This is especially the case for women.

In addition to providing formal services, governments also influence the care provided through employment regulations. No jurisdiction requires employers to provide "caregiver leave." However, some employment or labour standards legislations allow short-term and unpaid leave. While most collective agreements simply reflect the statutory emphasis on parental, sick and bereavement leave, some include additional leave provisions for those with disabilities and for personal reasons. The Public Service Alliance of Canada, for example, has negotiated leave with pay for family-related responsibilities. In this case, family is broadly defined to include not only spouses and common-law partners but also any of the children dependent on them. Parents as well as step-parents or foster parents are considered family and so are any relatives permanently residing in the employee's household or with whom the employee resides. The paid leave is only for a maximum of five days, although leave without pay is allowed for long-term care of a parent for up to five years (Treasury Board of Canada 2000).

Physical location also influences what care is provided, in part because formal services vary within provinces. Urban populations often have better access to care supports than do rural ones. "Poor quality housing and insufficient health and social services characterize many rural communities. Distance makes access to services more difficult and adversely affects rural women's ability to provide care" (Blakley and Jaffe 1999:3). Declining employment opportunities in rural areas, combined with health care reforms, mean fewer resources for increasing needs. This, in turn, means greater inequality in coping ability (Cloutier-Fisher and Joseph 2000) and Native communities in particular frequently lack formal, community based services (Buchignani and Armstrong-Esther 1999).

People living in large urban centres are more likely to find services that respond to their particular cultural or religious practices. For example, concentrated populations mean urban Japanese Canadians can access culturally sensitive programs. Such access can affect whether or not they use formal care services at all, regardless of need, and may matter as much as quality and location in seeking care (Chubachi 1999; Dorazio-Migliore 1999).

A person's physical location also matters in terms of informal caregiving. The further away friends, relatives and volunteers are, the more difficult it is to provide direct personal care. Children move away for education or employment; people emigrate, leaving behind their relatives. Nevertheless, many people do provide care-at-a-distance, especially care that is of the management sort (Rosenthal and Martin-Matthews 1999) or they move themselves or others in order to give care. In 1996, nearly half-a-million Canadians moved to give or receive care. The majority of those who moved were married, more than one-third had children under the age of fifteen in addition to their paid work. Although daughters are the most likely to make such moves, a significant proportion are friends (18 percent) or other relatives (Cranswick 1999). Living arrangements do not play a central role in emotional support and may be provided in person, by telephone, email or letter from anywhere, but living with someone may be the major determinant of help with activities of daily living; even more important than a marital or blood relationship (Chappell and Blandford 1991).

Social location matters at least as much as physical location in terms of what care is provided. Being a mother, daughter or spouse is critical, because daughters and mothers are the most common primary caregivers, followed by spouses, friends and volunteers (Frederick and Fast 1999; Campbell and Martin-Matthews 2000; Morris et al. 1999). We have little Canadian information on caregiving among same-sex couples or singles, but we do know that the gay and lesbian communities have formed support organizations and care services, especially for those suffering from HIV/AIDS (Taylor, forthcoming).

Gender and income profoundly influence what care is provided. According to a recent study, "Women family members were expected to supplement home care services without pay and at great personal expense in terms of their own health, incomes, benefits, career development and pension accumulation, while men were not under as much pressure to do so" (Morris et al. 1999:vi). Financial costs were picked up by recipients and families. Those without money simply do without and the poor or isolated fare worst of all. Deinstitutionalization, early discharge, day surgery and cutbacks in public health services all shift more care work and care costs onto individuals and families, particularly women. The more that care is privatized, the more the poor cannot afford it. Those without homes or relatives are particularly at risk of not receiving care (Fuller 2002; Willson and Howard 2002; Armstrong and Armstrong 2002; Bernier and Dallaire 2002; Gurevich 1999).

Finally, the needs of the person receiving care are a critical component in what care is provided. Those who are expected to recover after day surgery or early discharge from a hospital place high, immediate demands on caregivers for assistance in the full range of caregiving activities. Patients recovering from cardiac surgery, for example, require monitoring for their heart rate, for infection and for wound healing; they need reassurance and comfort, as well as help in eating, bathing, going to the toilet, keeping the house in order and in managing their diet and exercise program (King and Koop 1999). However, these demands are expected to diminish over time until care is eventually no longer required. The situation is quite different for someone suffering from Alzheimer's or multiple sclerosis. Care needs in these circumstances can only increase with time and will last until death.

Care, therefore, varies according to the stage of an illness. For example, initially cancer care may involve mainly management and emotional support. During and after treatment it may require the full range of care forms. If the cancer is treated successfully, the need for all but the emotional and social support may disappear. If the treatment fails, then care needs increase over a relatively short term and end with death.

Similarly, a chronic disease like multiple sclerosis, for example, may go into remission, allowing a person to live relatively independently for long periods. Arthritis and rheumatism may mean that only heavy housework and house maintenance are a problem for a long time, with more needs appearing over time. Stroke patients may recover fully after temporary severe disability, or become quite dependent for the rest of their lives (Stewart 2000).

Some chronic diseases and disabilities, however, exist from birth and mean that life is only possible with the provision of the full range of care, or with one form of care throughout life (The Roeher Institute 2001). Others may become paraplegic suddenly as a result of an accident. Care throughout life, or for most of it, is not uncommon. Of the fifty-three women interviewed for a study of rural caregivers, five had been caregiving for more than twenty years and one had been doing so for thirty-five years. Such caregivers provide care "all the time," often with little support from the formal system (Blakley and Jaffe 1999).

In short, what unpaid care is provided depends on government policies and on the health issue, as well as on physical and social location. Formal care does not substitute for informal care. Rather, most care is informal or self-care and supplemented by formal services.

Who Needs Care?

The short answer to this question is, "everyone" at least at some time in their lives. The surprising answer is, not necessarily seniors. According to a recent study based on Statistics Canada data, "when it comes to receiving assistance from others, similar proportions of seniors and non-seniors received assistance. And across age groups, only a minority reported that they received no assistance" (Keating et al. 1999:17). Another Statistics Canada report describes seniors as a diverse group that is aging well (Lindsay 1999). More than nine out of ten seniors live in a private household and, although over half say they have some help with household chores and personal tasks, half also say that they provide care to others (Lindsay 1999; Robb et al. 1999). In other words, for many seniors care is an exchange of services. Nevertheless, a significant number of seniors do need care. Of the 30 percent who required health-related personal assistance, three out of four needed assistance with daily living activities and one-quarter required extensive personal care. Women were not only more likely to need care, they were also more likely to have those needs go unmet. The lower the income and education, the greater the unmet need. Living alone also meant that the necessary care was less likely to be provided (Chen and Wilkins 1998). While most of the care is provided by informal caregivers, losing a partner is a major factor in entry into the use of formal home care services (Wilkins and Beaudet 2000).

The number of people with long-term disabilities is growing, and, like seniors, they are a diverse group. Their disabilities may be physical, mental or intellectual, or a combination of these; they may be life-long, result from a particular event or develop with age. The disability may mean only one form of care is required or it may mean the entire array of supports is necessary during one period or throughout life (The Roeher Institute 2001). For example, better care and better conditions for health mean that only now are many people with intellectual disabilities living to grow old. Many were originally placed in institutions but in recent years have moved into communities where they may no longer have family connections, or their families feel hesitation about taking on their care and guilt about placing them in an institution (Salvatori et al. 1998).

Shorter term, but often more intense care, is required by those with terminal illnesses and by those released early from hospital or undergoing day surgery. The increased demand for care after early release from hospital or day surgery strains existing community resources, often leaving the frail elderly who have been receiving care without much formal assistance (Cloutier-Fisher and Joseph 2000). Palliative care services are beginning to appear both as formal residential services and as support for informal caregivers in the home.

Who Provides Care?

The clear answer to the question is, women. As daughters, mothers, partners, friends, or volunteers, women are the overwhelming majority of unpaid primary caregivers and spend more time than men do in providing care. Women are much more likely than men to offer personal care and emotional support. Men's contributions are more likely to be concentrated in care management or household maintenance, shopping or transportation (Rosenthal and Martin-Matthews 1999; Campbell and Martin-Matthews 2000). In other words, women are more likely to provide the care that is daily and inflexible while men provide care that can be more easily planned and organized around paid work (Gignac et al. 1996). Men are also more likely than women to get formal help when they do provide care, on the assumptions that they must have paid jobs and that they lack the skills necessary to provide care (King and Koop 1999; Aronson and Neysmith 1997; Morris et al. 1999; Keefe and Fancey 1997). Yet women manage to provide personal care even when they have paid jobs, although higher income women may be able to become more care managers than care providers (Rosenthal and Martin-Matthews 1999). The little research available on differences among women caregivers suggests that income and education matter at least as much as culture in terms of the kinds and amounts of care provided (Chubahi 1999; Dorazio-Migliore 1999). While most women want to provide various kinds of informal care, they do not want to be "conscripted" into this relationship (National Forum on Health 1997:19). And the poorer women are, regardless of their culture, the more likely they are to have little choice about providing care (Morris et al. 1999).

Some men have provided, and continue to provide, the full range of care forms. Like women, they care for their spouses. However, fewer men are called on for such care because their wives usually outlive them – a result of women's greater longevity and the pattern of men marrying women significantly younger than themselves. Men also care for their parents, providing up to one-quarter of the care (Campbell and Martin-Matthews 2000). They care for their same-sex partners and serve as volunteers who manage care, provide transport and support, deliver meals and do household chores (McCann and Wadsworth

1992; Taylor forthcoming; Campbell and Martin-Matthews 2002). And like women, men may also provide care to siblings, in-laws or other relatives (Buchignani and Armstrong-Esther).

Friends also provide considerable caregiving, although we know less about them than we do about the spouses, mothers and children who are caregivers. A Statistics Canada study found that nearly one in five of those who had moved in order to provide care were friends rather than relatives, suggesting that some friends do much more than simply offer the occasional visit (Cranswick 1999).

We know even less about differences among caregivers related to culture. The research that does exist indicates no major differences in the provision of care but some in the stated commitment to care. For example, Japanese Canadians express a high commitment to filial obligation. This is reflected in the provision of emotional support but not in support through financial or other services (Kobayashi 2000). Some cultural groups are also much more likely than others to live in households that hold several generations, suggesting cross-generational caregiving. However, while East Indian immigrants, for example, tend to live in multi-generational households, it is important not to assume that this, like the lower use of formal services, simply indicates cultural choices. It may be as much about immigration regulations requiring support for sponsored relatives and limited economic resources as it is about preference (Dhawan 1998). That Chinese-, Greek- and Italian-origin seniors are less likely to live alone than are other Canadians may reflect low incomes, lack of pensions and immigration rules as much as cultural values (Brotman 1998). Similarly, the numbers of Native seniors living with relatives may reflect poverty as much as choice or values (Buchignani and Armstrong-Esther).

Like sponsored immigrants, spouses face rules governing support. The rules are fairly clear in terms of financial support, but less clear when it comes to providing direct care services. It is not evident that spousal support means you could take your partner to court to demand they change your diapers, insert your catheter or attach your oxygen mask. Certainly many of the policies and regulations in health care assume such support, especially from women, and enforce it through a failure to provide alternatives or through regulations. In Ontario, for example, government guidelines for in-home services say that people are not eligible for services until they have exhausted the support capacities of their family and friends, without any regard to whether the caregivers are employed or not (Armstrong and Armstrong 1999). Who constitutes a family for the purposes of providing such care, however, is not clear even in the regulations.

Children may face legal obligations for support of their parents. The filial responsibility laws require children to provide support if parents need support, have supported the children in the past and if the children can afford to provide support (Snell 1990; Bracci 2000). Sons are more likely, given higher wages, to be able to afford financial assistance. It is perhaps not surprising that these laws are seldom used, in part, because many sons do support their parents when they can, just as spouses and same-sex couples and friends do. When they cannot or when they reject their responsibility, the enforcement of these filial laws can undermine family relationships (Snell 1990; Bracci 2000).

Employees also have legal obligations, ones that may prevent rather than promote caregiving. One in four employees provide care and a large proportion of care providers are employed (MacBride-King 1999). Not surprisingly, those with both eldercare and child care responsibilities, most of whom are women, are the most likely to lose time at work as a result of caregiving (Cranswick 1999). The very limited leave allowed for such care, combined with very few protections from being fired when caregiver stress leads to missed time at their paid jobs, mean that caregivers are very vulnerable at work. Those who care for people unrelated by blood or marriage may be particularly at risk.

CARE AND CONSEQUENCES

Although caregiving and care receiving are about relationships, much of the research on the impact of caregiving has focused on the negative consequences for providers, viewing care recipients as objects rather than as participating subjects. Not surprisingly, caregiver burden is a common theme in the literature.

There are many and varied aspects to the burden of caregiving. Rural women who provide care describe feeling frustrated, especially with the repetitiveness of the tasks and the problem of dealing with the frustration of the care recipient (Blakley and Jaffe 1999). They have to convince their husbands to allow them to bathe them and, like others who care for younger adults with severe physical disabilities, describe the "difficult and potentially hazardous situations resulting from a combination of the weight of the person being bathed and the lack of strength of both parties" (Gutman 1995:26). Lack of training for what is highly skilled caregiving also creates additional stress on relationships. For many caregivers, the most emotionally upsetting activities are those related to bladder and bowel management, in part because they are such intimate tasks. Male caregivers found bathing their wives disturbing for similar reasons (Gutman 1995). Rural caregivers feel ineffective in dealing with mood swings of the care recipient and with their own guilt: guilt about being healthy, guilt about not understanding the illness and guilt about not making the right choices for the care recipient (Blakley and Jaffe 1999). Such guilt is widely shared among caregivers, especially by the women who provide most of the care. It may be compounded by their role as sole confidante and decision-maker and by cultural pressures (Dorazio-Migliore 1999). Caregivers who move to provide care, like those who live-in or live close-by, report changes in their sleep patterns, a decline in overall health, depression, a reduction in their social activities and holidays, and extra expenses (Cranswick 1999). A study of caregivers for those with Parkinson's suggests that the strain is greater the closer the caregiver is to the recipient (Moore 1997). In other words, loving the recipient may make it more difficult.

Stress of all sorts is a recurring theme, as are family conflicts over who provides care and what kind of care is required. Conflicts may arise between informal and formal caregivers, over what care should be provided and how it should be provided. Moreover, shifting care to homes means that formal services invade the household and "boundaries separating these domains" are continually crossed, creating greater strain on the entire household (Ward-Griffin 1998). New policy initiatives urge partnerships between families and paid providers, but this may well be more of an exploitative relationship than a partnership one, especially if the primary purpose is the reduction of public expenditure. In the partnership, "most family caregivers were left socially isolated without adequate resources to provide care. Intentionally or not, holding family caregivers accountable for the provision of care without adequate resources is completely unacceptable." Indeed, the research, on nurse/family relationships warns that "failure to provide resources to help family members provide care could risk even further increases in health costs, as injuries or illness" result for caregivers. Moreover, "failure to provide resources to help family members provide care could risk even further increases in health care costs, as injuries or illnesses of the elder and/or family caregiver ensue" (Ward-Griffin and McKeever 2000:101). Privacy is reduced for the entire household and for their relationships. Even before the most recent cutbacks in services, research indicated that caregivers have higher rates of affective and anxiety disorders than non-caregivers and that they use mental health services twice as much (Cochrane et al. 1997). Caregivers for people with dementia are particularly at risk, and among those, people whose first language is neither English nor French are especially fragile (Meshefedjian et al. 1998). Immigrants may feel particularly isolated and limited in their access to services that meet their needs (Dhawan 1998). This may contribute to depression, with those who have no outside help suffering the most (Dhawan 1998).

Effects on Caregivers

Caregiving can mean career interruption, time lost from work, financial loss and, especially for women, even job loss (Statistics Canada 1997). Indeed, women feel much greater tension than men between their caregiving and their paid work, and between their caregiving and other family responsibilities. This is not surprising, given that women do more of the personal care and domestic work (Gignac et al. 1996; Rosenthal and Martin-Matthews 1999). For both women and men, the consequences of such interruptions can be felt far into the future in terms of low pensions and benefits in their own old age.

Although friends and volunteers also provide considerable caregiving, virtually all the caregiving burden research has been done on relatives, especially on the mothers, wives and daughters who do the majority of the care. This lack of research may not simply reflect a failure to recognize non-family members' contributions, however. It may also reflect the fact that friends and volunteers have more choice about where and when they provide care, as well as about what care they provide. Similarly, there is a lack of research on same-sex partners, but there is little reason to believe the burden would be any lighter for them.

There is considerable discussion in the literature about the subjective factors, such as negative attitudes and cultural values towards caregiving, that influence the impact on the caregiver. However, "a belief one is ill-equipped to meet the demands of caregiving may not be unrealistic. Economic factors, a lack of instrumental support or caregiver illness may greatly impede one's ability to cope and may thus be a realistic, objective perception" (O'Rourke et al. 1996):592. In other words, caregivers may perceive a burden because there generally is one. This is especially the case for those who must provide long-term and constant care (Echenberg 1998).

It should be emphasized, however, that caregiving also brings rewards. Caregivers experience warmth and satisfaction; they get joy from helping others and often feel rewarded through the personal interaction and the very real support they often receive in return (MacBride-King 1999). Yet, like most human relationships, caregivers' experiences are contradictory (Aronson 1998). Resentment, stress, frustration and ill health too often occur along with the good parts, and are most likely to occur in the absence of support, relief and choice. The strain is too often manifested as abuse (Spencer et al. 1996) not only of the elderly but also of the disabled, whatever their age. Older people with intellectual disabilities may be doubly disadvantaged by prejudice against both the elderly and the disabled. Support groups, while often offered as an inexpensive way to relieve the burden of caregiving, have little impact, especially in the absence of other, more material, supports (Lavoie 1995; Colantonio et al. 1998).

Effects on Care Recipients

What about the burden on care recipients? We know less about this burden or about their views on the relationship. What we do know suggests that they too have burdens in addition to those caused by their physical or mental problems or both, especially when their low incomes and cutbacks in services eliminate choices about care. Care receivers may be placed in a position of "compulsory acquiescence," not primarily by their informal care providers but rather by the public system's failure to offer them choices (Aronson 1990). Elderly women experience conflicts between their need for support and the expectation of self-sufficiency, as well as between the media panic over the costs of an aging population and the system's failure to recognize the specificity of their individual needs (Aronson 1990). Seeking to maintain reciprocity and their pride, these women feel the strain of limiting their demands and the strain within their relationships (Aronson 1990). Like caregivers, they experience guilt and frustration (Aronson 1998). On the other hand, having a partner can make a significant difference, even in ill health. Indeed, "married seniors in poor health enjoy a high level of emotional support and are just as socially engaged as those in good health" (Crompton and Kemeny 1999:26). It seems likely this is the case with couples or others who are not married but who have enjoyed a long life together. As is the case with caregivers, there appear to be significant differences between the burdens felt by women and those felt by men. "Female respondents described feeling guilty when their husbands did laundry and prepared meals if they had never been involved in these tasks before." At the same time, these women with osteoarthritis or osteoporosis defined spousal help with mobility, at home or in the community, as simply part of the relationship. Men, on the other hand, did not usually see help from a spouse with such household tasks or with personal care as dependence (Cott and Gignac). In other words, the work becomes invisible when either gender does non-traditional tasks.

In sum, caring is about complex relationships that take a wide variety of forms. These relationships are shaped not simply by individuals, their culture and their personal histories but also by the services, supports and alternatives available to them. The focus in recent research has been on the caregiver in part because the conditions for caregiving are changing significantly, and changing in ways that make caregiving more difficult and varied. "Those with more resources, by virtue of class, race or age, will be better able to offset the costs of caring, whether by purchasing private help or by being able to negotiate public resources from a more privileged position" (Aronson and Neysmith 1997:51). And those in stable relationships supported by adequate income and services are in the best position to give and receive care.

THE CONTEXT FOR CAREGIVING: ONE HUNDRED YEARS

Context matters. It shapes the possibilities for caregiving, setting the stage for patterns in care. Much of the discussion about caregiving, however, is based on myths about the past and the present. Such myths often distort our assessment of legislative, regulatory and policy options, so it is important to look at what has and has not changed much over the last hundred years.

What Has Not Changed Significantly Over the Last Hundred Years

Neither government fears that families will shirk their responsibilities for care nor fears of an aging population are new, although neither fear has much justification. One hundred years ago the majority of seniors lived in private households and were listed as family heads or spouses of family heads, indicating relative economic and social self-sufficiency (Montigny and Chambers 1998). This is still the case today, with most of the aged living with spouses and only a minority listed as dependent on others. Over 90 percent of seniors now live in a private household, most with their immediate family (Lindsay 1999). At the same time, living in extended families is not uncommon today. Indeed, the number of three-generation households increased in the last decade of the twentieth century, with half of them headed by immigrants and 40 percent including someone with some disability (Che-Alford and Hamm 1999).

Previously, like today, many adult children continued to live with their parents because they could not find paid work that would support them in living independent lives (Dillon 1998). The elderly were most likely to live with their children in rural areas while overcrowding and poverty in urban areas made co-residency much less likely (Struthers 1994). Although co-residence may well mean that adult children provide some care for their elderly parents, it also often means that they themselves receive support. In both periods, women without spouses were more likely than men to live with their children because they did not have enough income to live on their own (Montigny 1997). Such women were likely to be contributing members of the household, especially in rural areas, and not simply dependent care recipients (Montigny 1997).

Even though the elderly were and are mainly self-sufficient, concern about the costs of an aging population recurs throughout the century. The end of the nineteenth century, like the end of the twentieth, saw the "rapid increase in demand for institutional accommodation for the province's aged population during a period of fiscal restraint" while governments blamed families for shirking responsibilities. A century ago, 3 percent of the elderly and of those with disabilities lived in institutions while about 1 percent do so today (Montigny 1997:89; see also Davies, forthcoming).

The government response then, like now, was to restrict admission to institutions and argue that care was a family obligation, but some families were not able or willing to provide support and providing it often caused conflicts within families. The recognition of such conflicts can be found historically in the "elaborate provisions in wills and maintenance agreements" obliging support (Elliott, forthcoming). Similarly, filial laws first introduced in Quebec in 1866 indicate that children did not always support their parents in their old age, although the limited cases of actual enforcement of these laws suggest either that most children provided support or that parents were unwilling to force the case (Guest 1980). Governments also began as early as 1906 to discuss pensions for the elderly and other forms of support for the disabled because many of the elderly and disabled did not have families providing care (Guest 1980).

Despite considerable evidence that support for those needing care has long been recognized as a collective and public responsibility (Davies, forthcoming; McDaniel and Lewis 1998) even stronger evidence indicates state commitment to and enforcement of family responsibility (Snell 1996). Yet in both periods, there is little evidence to support the claim that many families abandon their responsibilities for the elderly and the younger disabled or that age alone creates dependency. Most families, then and now, care for their kin. Marriage vows once involved spouses promising to love, honour and obey in sickness and in health, and this is still the expectation today whether or not such vows are involved. Equally important, concerns about an aging population are not new and such concerns persist even in the face of evidence indicating that the overwhelming majority of the elderly do not rely on the state for care. Indeed, many of the elderly themselves provide care in ways that relieve the state of care costs.

Charities and volunteers have not abandoned their responsibilities during the twentieth century either. At the end of the nineteenth century, governments like the one in Ontario "came to accept a great deal of responsibility for the care of the ill, the insane, the destitute, and the dependent aged" (Montigny 2000:74). At the same time, much of this care was provided through the funding of charitable or lay organizations. This is still the case today. Canadians also continue to volunteer in large numbers, through both formal and informal networks to deliver food and to transport people to care services, to provide information, to visit, to offer personal support and care (Chappell and Prince 1997; Hall and Statistics Canada 1998). "One-fifth of caregivers were neighbours and friends, evidence that the caring society also reaches beyond family obligations" (Keating et al. 1999:53). Moreover, volunteers now do a considerable amount of caregiving that would otherwise be done by paid workers, "transformed into wageless workers with less control over their caring work" (Esteves 2000:154).

The notion that families and charities provided all the care desired, and did it so well, is often linked to the notion of everyone living in large, rural households based on a heterosexual couple still with the same partner they married in their teens. Yet households were much more diverse than that. Women and men often waited until they had the economic resources to marry and a significant number never married at all. Death from childbirth, from injury, from infectious diseases and other illnesses meant that many heterosexual couples found themselves widowed early. Remarriage, and along with it the blending of households, was common. While the law made divorce difficult, desertion was not uncommon and there is every reason to believe that the deserters and deserted later took up residence with others, usually without the benefit of marriage. Nor was it unknown for friends to live together. What is not known is how many of these friends were also sexual partners. Urban households, especially those that were not affluent, tended to be quite small (Parr 1995). Urban households were also much more likely to contain recent immigrants who usually occupied areas of the city recently abandoned by other immigrants only to be replaced themselves by the next wave of immigration (Porter 1965). In some areas, such as B.C., there were far more men than women and the men often looked after and lived with each other (Davies, forthcoming). In other areas, like Paris, Ontario, women formed the primary labour force and provided important support networks for each other (Davies, forthcoming; Bailey 2000; Eichler 2000; Smart 2000; Parr 1990; Bradbury 1993).

Nor can it be assumed that all families were based on a mother at home with time to care for others while father earned the bread needed by the entire household. In rural areas, most women worked hard in production on the farm and had little spare time for caregiving. In urban areas, many men did not earn enough to support the family and the entire household entered the labour force. For those who were not married, paid work was often the only option. However, that paid work frequently involved providing care in someone else's home. In fact, the household with a male breadwinner earning enough income to support the family and with a woman who had enough time to provide care was a dominant family form only for a brief period following World War II. It was a form made possible both by high, secure and well-paid male employment and by a welfare state that offered not only considerable support but also a redistribution of economic resources (Bradbury 1993; Cohen 1988).

What Has Changed Significantly Over the Last Hundred Years?

While there are very similar patterns in some areas over the last century, there are also some quite radical differences that create different conditions and demands for care.

One of the most obvious changes is health. Better nutrition, transportation, working and housing conditions, along with more formal education, have all contributed to better health. At the beginning of the twentieth century, Canadians were not generally in good health and even the Sickness Survey of 1950-51 showed that "Canadians were not a healthy people" (Taylor 1978:5). Relatively secure employment and decent wages for many men and some women made an important difference to the health not only of the men but also of those who were largely dependent on them. So did the welfare state. Much of the planning in the aftermath of World War II was based on the assumption that "organized provision will be made in the post-war world for the risks and contingencies of family life that are beyond the capacity of most of them to finance adequately from their own resources" (Marsh 1975:7).

Under the welfare state, income tax was changed to make those with higher incomes pay a greater share. This progressive taxation strategy contributed to a redistribution of resources. Labour standards legislation and workers' compensation protected many workers, as did unemployment insurance, maternity leave and both public and private job-related pension schemes. Unionization became easier and more effective in gaining rights for workers. Human Rights legislation supported equity in a variety of situations and allowed affirmative action in others. The universal pension for elderly people reduced poverty and dependence in old age, while the Canada Assistance Plan, the means-tested Guaranteed Income Supplement linked to the Old Age Pension and various plans for those with disabilities all helped reduce inequality and improve health (Guest 1980; Banting 1982; McGilly 1991; Echenberg 1998; The Roeher Institute 2001). More public transport made more people mobile and public housing gave some a home. Innovations in housing strategies for the elderly and the disabled helped many live with dignity without depending on their families (Blackie et al. 1985; Gutman and Blackie 1988; Doyle 1989; Gutman 1989; Canada Mortgage and Housing Corporation 1983). Universal public education from kindergarten to high school also contributed to greater equality and thus to health (Banting 1982; Guest 1980; Myles 2000). Unlike most of the support in the nineteenth century, many of these programs were defined as rights of citizenship rather than as charity schemes targeted at the deserving (Armstrong 1997).

Together, and combined with the move from primary resources and goods production to services and the accompanying urbanization, these welfare state measures contributed to a significant decline in the time men spent in the labour force. At the beginning of the century, men began paid work at an early age, worked long hours, had few or no vacations and stayed working until they were no longer physically able, often gradually reducing paid work and dying shortly after they finally quit (Chappell et al. 1986). Now full-time paid employment cannot begin at least until age sixteen, and for most it begins far later, after years of formal education. For many it ends at least at age sixty-five, where compulsory retirement is legal, and pensions or early retirement packages mean some people leave even before then. Most men can then expect to live well beyond retirement from their paid work. However, this development may have contradictory effects on men and the extent to which they enjoy being out of the labour force will depend in part on both what kind of job they leave and what kind of income they have.

Public health measures such as immunization, food inspection, drug regulation and water treatment reduced the spread of infectious and other diseases. Universal health care coverage for hospitals and doctors were part of this welfare state development, as were the expansion of residential care facilities and public home care services. Universal coverage, combined with new developments in drugs and techniques, were major factors in falling infant and maternal mortality rates, as well as in the successful treatment of many illnesses (Armstrong and Armstrong 1998). By the 1990s, the overwhelming majority of Canadians rated their health as good to excellent – even among those over age seventy-five – and Canada was near the top on most health indicators Rosenberg and Moore 1997). Many more people survived with significant or severe disabilities and with chronic diseases. Those with intellectual disabilities, for example, are finally living into old age (Salvatori et al. 1998). Old age also became older as longevity increased. Nearly 12 percent of the population was over sixty-five in 1999 and those over eighty-five are the fastest growing segment. Women are the overwhelming majority of the old old (Ontario Human Rights Commission 2000).

Of course, the welfare state was far from perfect and far from successful in eliminating inequality. Many more men than women were able to benefit from the employment-related schemes and few with long-term disabilities had access to these rights-based schemes Echenberg 1998). Welfare programs often served to reinforce dependency without alleviating poverty and offered support as charity. Nevertheless, contributions of the welfare state to reducing inequality have become increasingly clear as its demise coincides with growing inequality among both individuals and families (Armstrong 1997; McDaniel 1997; Yalnizyan 1998; Davies et al. 2001; Sauve 1999; Allahan and Cote 1998). Virtually all of these programs are under threat or have been reduced or transformed into targeted programs. Meanwhile new problems are emerging, the most obvious of which are HIV/AIDS and Alzheimer's.

One program in particular under threat is the health care system. Enormous changes have taken place in this system throughout the last hundred years but the last decade has seen some of the most important for caregiving. New techniques, drugs and technologies have made it possible to do day surgery and provide many other interventions on an outpatient basis or with shorter patient stays. Moreover, many of the sophisticated treatments once available only within hospitals can now be done at home, thanks in part to new equipment.

Combined with an emphasis on cost-cutting, these developments mean that many people are sent out of hospital while still requiring complex and skilled care. The obvious consequence is more informal caregiving and unpaid caregivers providing much more complex care. The less obvious consequence is the entry into the home of strangers to assess the need for, and to provide, care. This can mean less privacy and more conflict over what care is provided by whom (Armstrong and Armstrong 1996). Perhaps least obvious is the shifting of care costs onto the caregiver or recipient and their often shared concern about the quality of care provided by informal carers. It must be emphasized that this is not care being sent back home, where it was once done by mothers and daughters. Our grandmothers never cleaned catheters or checked intravenous tubes, they did not examine incisions or do much wound care.

Little research exists on this new form of care but what is available indicates that the caregiving is done primarily by women. For elderly patients discharged early from hospital, access to formal in-home services were significant in boosting morale, perhaps in part because they had confidence in the skills of the provider (Chambers et al. 1990). In the case of patients recovering from cardiac surgery, eighty-four percent of the women caregivers were employed outside the home. Their jobs in "lower status positions" mean that leaves are difficult to obtain and caregiving, even for a short period, could threaten their jobs (King and Koop 1999).

The other relatively recent development in health care is the move of people from institutions into the community. Deinstitutionalization began with psychiatric patients in the late 1960s (Simmons 1990) and now applies to all those previously cared for in large facilities. Then, like now, the move has often been made without appropriate alternatives available and the "community" often means a poorly-equipped home or the street (Layton 2000). Those at home are expected to provide care, and the expectations are higher for women. Moreover, such care often means giving up paid employment, and women are more likely than men to leave the labour force to provide care, in part because they have the lower paying jobs (Statistics Canada 2000). It may simply make sense, at least in the short term, for the lowest paid member to leave the labour force in order to provide necessary care and few jobs allow women to take paid leave to provide care.

This leads directly to a major change in women's labour force participation. Today, unlike a century ago, most women are in the labour force for most of their adult years (Statistics Canada 2000). They have jobs for many reasons, including the fact that jobs grew in traditional female work with the expansion of the welfare state. However, the single most important reason for taking paid work is the same for women as for men: they need the income (Armstrong and Armstrong 1994; The Vanier Institute of the Family). Although women have made significant progress within the labour force, they are still segregated into the lowest paid occupations. They are also over-represented in part-time and temporary work. Those who are self-employed seldom have people working for them and many hold multiple jobs (Statistics Canada 2000). Moreover, women's steady improvement since the 1950s seems to have halted or even reversed. In 1999, 41 percent of employed women aged 15 to 64 had a non-standard employment arrangement, compared to 35 percent in 1989, and women's labour force participation rates have stayed virtually the same for the last decade (Statistics Canada 2000). In that same year, 3 percent of women, compared to 1 percent of men, in full-time jobs lost time at work because of family responsibilities (Statistics Canada 2000). The increases in women's non-standard work may in part be explained by their increasing caregiving activities. Instead of losing time at work, they may have to take jobs that require less time or that can be done at home. Women's full-time work is less likely than men's to come with a private pension and non-standard work is even less likely to have any benefits at all. As a result, many of the women who account for the majority of the elderly have only public pensions. And for many, the lack of a pension is a direct result of their caregiving (Townson and Canadian Advisory Council on the Status of Women 1995).

At the same time, many employment protections have been removed in a deregulated market, leaving fewer and fewer households with even one secure, decently paid job to support the household. Partly in response to these changes, more men and women are working longer hours, often at two jobs (Statistics Canada 2000). As a result, fewer and fewer families have the time or resources to provide much care just as care demands are increasing. This seems like a volatile mix.

There have also been changes in family patterns. There are fewer marriages and fewer children born closer together in terms of age within marriages. Openly common-law relationships have become much more common, as have openly gay and lesbian relationships. More marriages end in divorce and more blended families have children who still have other living parents outside the current marriage (Ambert 1998). More families have only one parent, most often a mother. Housing and job shortages, as well as inadequate incomes, are forcing more people to live with relatives and friends. And new patterns of immigration mean that households are much more culturally and racially diverse (Woolley 1998). What these developments mean for caregiving is difficult to determine but it is clear that the changes in relationships will influence where, when and how care can or will be provided. And it seems likely that there are fewer and fewer family members, and thus fewer people, to provide that care.

The Changes That Matter For Care

What this summary indicates is that people have provided, and continue to provide, care for friends, relatives and strangers. For the most part, they do it willingly and with care (Wolfson et al. 1993). Moreover, those who receive care now or in the past themselves provide care, and caregiving is often part of rewarding relationships. However, the demands on caregivers are expanding enormously with the increasing acuity and disability levels of those receiving informal care. Longevity is also contributing to the workload, although not as much as public discourse would suggest. Moreover, there are more people needing this complex care at the same time as the welfare state is reducing the services provided in the formal system and increasing pressures on families in general and women in particular to fill the gaps. Yet more and more women have little choice but to work in the labour force. Few of their labour force jobs allow them to provide care and, if they do give up full-time paid work in order to care, they jeopardize not only their future employment but also their money for old age (Morris et al. 1999). More and more research suggests that this caregiving is often a burden under current conditions, placing strains not only on the health of the providers and recipients but also on their relationships and on their current and future finances.

FRAMEWORK FOR ASSESSING LEGISLATION, REGULATION AND POLICY

This summary of one hundred years of caregiving provides a basis for developing a framework for assessing government intervention. Legislation, regulation and social policy should seek to facilitate caregiving among adults and to do so in ways that allow both care providers and care recipients to retain their dignity and their relationships. This means asking the following questions:

1. *Are caregiving and care receiving voluntary?* Caregiving can be voluntary only if there is access to alternatives and if there are the kinds of supports available that allow choices to be made. This, in turn, can mean the most effective and efficient care. The Hall Commission (Canada 1964) which provided the basis for public health care recommended that a full range of services, including home care, long-term care and pharmacare, be publicly provided on the grounds that this would help ensure that services were delivered not only appropriately and in an accessible manner but also in the least expensive manner because choice would be based more on need than simply on what was available.

2. *Can caregiving be equally shared among women and men?* Women told the National Forum on Health, a body established by Prime Minister Chrétien to advise on the future of health care, that they did not want to be "conscripted" (National Forum on Health 1997:19) into unpaid caregiving. The research clearly shows that such caregiving is, and has been, primarily women's work. This is the case regardless of age, income, labour force participation, cultural, physical or legal locations. While the values of the women who provide care play some role in this workload, there is significant evidence to demonstrate that legislation, regulations and policy construct women as caregivers.

3. *Can caregiving be culturally sensitive without making inappropriate assumptions about cultural groups and without contravening other equity principles?* Equity, if defined as exactly the same services provided to everyone, can mean services that do not respond to many people's specific needs. Experience with both the *Canada Health Act* and the *Canadian Human Rights Act* has shown that it is possible to establish principles that allow for considerable variety in how these principles are met. There is

considerable diversity in the needs, resources and desires of caregivers and recipients that should be, when appropriate, accommodated in legislation.

4. *Can the assumptions made about personal relationships related to caregiving be justified?* Legislation, regulations and policy often assume the heterosexual nuclear family. They also often assume that the women in particular in such families have the skills, resources, time and desire to provide care. Yet many people do not live in such relationships, and those that do may not see their families as the best place to find or give care. Equally important, caregiving often involves many people with no blood or marital ties who nevertheless need supports in order to provide care.

5. *Is there recognition of the different interests that need to be balanced in caregiving?* In searching for ways to facilitate caregiving, it is necessary to recognize that there are tensions and differences that can never be resolved but rather need to be balanced and understood in their particular contexts. Perhaps the most critical of these is the tension between care providers and care recipients. Each has different, and often contradictory, needs. Paid and unpaid providers also frequently have conflicting practices and agendas. So too do governments and institutions focused on cost saving when they encounter caregivers seeking supports. There are also tensions between the desire for privacy and the need for caregivers to share information, and between the transfer of care to the private home and the regular entry into that home of care providers. All these, and more, tensions exist within the larger one between individual and collective responsibility for care.

6. *Is need defined in ways that exclude some groups while privileging or stigmatizing others?* Programs and supports defined as welfare rather than as universal rights can serve to create inequalities. As the discussions and research that led to many social programs in Canada make clear, we are all at risk of illness and disability, and thus in need of care. Illness is usually not the fault of the individual and frail old age is seldom attributable to individual actions. Canadians have agreed that we have a collective responsibility for care and that care is a right, not a privilege. It is important for legislation, regulations and policy to reflect this right.

7. *What are the long term consequences?* Although some services, supports and obligations may seem to make sense today, they may have negative consequences in the future. So, for example, a woman who provides care for her partner may benefit immediately from a caregiver allowance but this allowance may mean she drops out of the labour force and finds herself in poverty when she is old. Moreover, the care she provides today may cut her off from friends who will provide her with support tomorrow. In thinking about consequences, we need to think beyond the provider and recipients to their network of relationships and to the larger society.

8. *Are the objectives reinforced or undermined by other legislation, regulations or policy?* Strategies in one sector may enable caregiving while those in another may mean caregiving is a burden. For example, flexible hours in paid work may allow women to be caregivers at home or in their community

but they may also serve to reinforce women's responsibility for this caregiving, limiting their capacity to do their paid work or threatening their health. Or respite services available for caregivers may be out of reach because there is no accessible public transit to the care. Or housing policies may mean that people who need some care cannot afford to live in their own homes or independently.

9. *Are the contributions of care recipients recognized and the skills required for giving care acknowledged?* While the research shows that care recipients are often the most vulnerable and in need of complex services, it also shows that many care recipients are themselves contributors in forms of caregiving. It is important to recognize their participation and facilitate it. It is just as important to recognize that care is skilled work, especially as more and more complex care needs are sent home.

10. *Are current patterns themselves constructs of policy or does policy reflect actual preferences and practices?* It is important to ask if policies have created patterns that are then replicated in ways that exclude alternatives. For example, current immigration laws on family unification mean that those families that want to live with relatives are the most likely to apply and, in any case, the regulations require these families to continue supporting the relatives brought into Canada under these provisions. It cannot be assumed that families who immigrate under such conditions reflect all families from these cultures, however, or that these families have the resources necessary to provide such care.

CONCLUDING REMARKS

The research on unpaid caregiving suggests "the need to refocus attention away from the creation of partnerships and protecting against unnecessary substitution towards broader concerns with supporting the partnerships that already exists" (Penning 2000:76). The risk is not that families will not provide care but rather that they will not be able to provide care without risking their health and their relationships if formal services fail to support them. Indeed, "more generous social programs reinforce both family and social responsibility" (Baker 1996:3). Under conditions of declining public support, broader definitions of family may simply mean more people are conscripted into care rather than better caregiving or better relationships. Without formal supports for unpaid caregiving, both the caregivers and their relationships are increasingly likely to fall apart. And such supports need to recognize the diversity in needs and the diversity in networks, networks that extend beyond kin to create the most satisfying care (Stewart 2000).

An earlier and longer version of this chapter was prepared for the Law Commission of Canada. The views expressed are those of the authors and do not necessarily reflect the views of the Commission. The accuracy of the information is solely the responsibility of the authors.

References

Allahan, A.L. and J.E. Cote. (1998). *Richer and Poorer: The Structure of Inequality in Canada.* Toronto: Lorimer.

Ambert, A.-M. (1998). *Divorce: Facts, Figures and Consequences.* Ottawa: The Vanier Institute of the Family.

Armstrong, P. (1997). "The Welfare State as History," in R.B. Blake, P. Bryden and J.F. Strain, (eds.), *The Welfare State in Canada: Past, Present and Future.* Concord, ON: Irwin Publishers.

Armstrong, P. and H. Armstrong. (1994). *The Double Ghetto: Canadian Women and Their Segregated Work* (third ed.). Toronto: Oxford University Press.

―――― (1998). *Universal Health Care: What the U.S. Can Learn from the Canadian Experience.* New York: New Press.

―――― (1996). *Wasting Away: The Undermining of Canadian Health Care.* Toronto: Oxford University Press.

―――― (2002). "Women, Privatization and Health Care Reform: The Ontario Case," in Pat Armstrong et al., *Exposing Privatization: Women and Health Care Reform in Canada.* Aurora: Garamond Press.

Aronson, J. (1990). "Old Women's Experiences of Needing Care: Choice or Compulsion?" *Canadian Journal on Aging/La Revue Canadienne du Vieillissement* 9 (3).

―――― (1998). "Women's Perspectives on Informal Care of the Elderly: Public Ideology and Personal Experience of Giving and Receiving Care," in D. Coburn, C. D'Arcy and G.M. Torrance (eds.), *Health and Canadian Society: Sociological Perspectives.* Toronto: University of Toronto Press.

Aronson, J. and S. Neysmith. (1997). "The Retreat of the State and Long-Term Provision: Implementations for Frail Elderly People, Unpaid Family Carers and Paid Home Care Workers." *Studies in Political Economy* 53 (Summer).

Bacovsky, R. (1997). *Federal, Provincial and Territorial Government Sponsored Drug Plans and Drug Databases: Background Information Prepared for the Conference on National Approaches to Pharmacare.*

Bailey, M. (2000). "Foreword." *Canadian Journal of Family Law* 17 (1).

Baker, M. (1996). *Reinforcing Obligations and Responsibilities between Generations: Policy Options from Cross-National Comparisons.* Ottawa: The Vanier Institute of the Family.

Banting, K.G. (1982). *The Welfare State and Canadian Federalism.* Kingston: Brown and Martin.

Bernier, J. and M. Dallaire, (2002). "What Price Have Women Paid for Health Care Reform? The Situation in Quebec," in Pat Armstrong et al., *Exposing Privatization: Women and Health Care Reform in Canada.* Aurora: Garamond Press.

Blackie, N.K., G.M. Gutman, Canadian Association on Gerontology, et al. (1985). *Innovations in Housing and Living Arrangements for Seniors.* Burnaby, BC: Gerontology Research Centre, Simon Fraser University.

Bracci, C. (2000). "Ties That Bind: Ontario's *Filial Responsibility Act.*" *Canadian Journal of Family Law* 17 (2).

Bradbury, B. (1993). *Working Families: Age, Gender and Daily Survival in Industrializing Montreal.* Toronto: McClelland and Stewart.

Brotman, S. (1998). "The Incidence of Poverty Among Seniors in Canada: Exploring the Impact of Gender, Ethnicity and Race." *Canadian Journal on Aging/La Revue Canadienne du Vieillissement* 17 (2).

Buchignani, N. and C. Armstrong-Esther. (1999). "Informal Care and Older Native Canadians." *Aging and Society* 19 (1):3-32.

Campbell, L.D. and A. Martin-Matthews. (2000). "Caring Sons: Exploring Men's Involvement in Filial Care." *Canadian Journal on Aging/La Revue Canadienne du Vieillissement* 1 (Spring).

Canada. (1964). *Report of the Royal Commission on Health Services (Hall Royal Commission).* Ottawa: Queen's Printer.

Canada Mortgage and Housing Corporation. (1983). *Housing the Elderly.* Ottawa: Canada Mortgage and Housing Corporation.

Canadian Home Care Association (in collaboration with L'Association des CLSC et des CHSLD du Quebec). (1998). *Portrait of Canada: An Overview of Public Home Care Programs.* Ottawa: Health Canada.

Chambers, L., P. Tugwell, C.H. Goldsmith, et al. (1990). "Impact of Home Care on Recently Discharged Elderly Hospital Patients in an Ontario Community." *Canadian Journal on Aging/La Revue Canadienne du Vieillissement* 9 (4).

Chappell, N. and A. Blandford. (1991). "Informal and Formal Care: Exploring the Complementarity." *Aging and Society* Vol. 11 (Part 3).

Chappell, N.L. and M.J. Prince. (1997). "Reasons Why Canadian Seniors Volunteer." *Canadian Journal on Aging/La Revue Canadienne du Vieillissement* 16 (2).

Chappell, N.L., L.A. Strain and A.A. Blandford. (1986). *Aging and Health Care: A Social Perspective.* Toronto: Holt Rinehart and Winston of Canada.

Che-Alford, J. and B. Hamm. (1999). "Under One Roof: Three Generations Living Together." *Canadian Social Trends* (Summer).

Chen, J. and R. Wilkins. (1998). "Seniors' Needs for Health-Related Personal Assistance." *Health Reports* 10 (11).

Chubachi, N. (1999). *Geographies of Nisei Japanese Canadians and Their Attitudes Towards Elderly Long-Term Care.* M.A., Kingston, ON: Queen's University.

Cloutier-Fisher, D. and A.E. Joseph. (2000). "Long-Term Care Restructuring in Rural Ontario: Retrieving Community Service User and Provider Narratives." *Social Science and Medicine* 50 (7-8).

Cochrane, J.J., P.N. Goering and J.M. Rogers. (1997). "The Mental Health of Informal Caregivers in Ontario: An Epidemiological Survey." *American Journal of Public Health* 87 (12).

Cohen, M.G. (1988). *Women's Work, Markets, and Economic Development in Nineteenth-Century Ontario.* Toronto, Buffalo: University of Toronto Press.

Colantonio, A., C. Cohen and S. Corlett. (1998). "Support Needs of Elderly Caregivers of Persons with Dementia." *Canadian Journal on Aging/La Revue Canadienne du Vieillissement* 17 (3).

Connidis, I.A. (1983). "Living Arrangement Choices of Older Residents." *Canadian Journal of Sociology/Cahiers canadiens de sociologie,* 8.

Cott, C.A. and M.A.M. Gignac. (DATE ????) "Independence and Dependence for Older Adults with Osteoarthritis or Osteoporosis." *Canadian Journal on Aging/La Revue Canadienne du Vieillissement* 18 (1).

Cranswick, K. (1999). "Help Close at Hand: Relocating to Give or Receive Care." *Canadian Social Trends* (Winter).

Crompton, S. and A. Kemeny. (1999). "In Sickness and in Health: The Well-Being of Married Seniors." *Canadian Social Trends* (Winter).

Dalley, G. (1988). *Ideologies of Caring: Rethinking Community and Collectivism.* Basingstoke, UK: Macmillan Education.

Davies, L., J.A. McMullin, W.R. Avison, et al. (2001). *Social Policy, Gender Inequality and Poverty.* Ottawa: Status of Women in Canada.

Davies, M.J. (Forthcoming). *Into the House of the Old: A History of Residential Care in B.C.* Unpublished Manuscript.

Denton, M. (1997). "The Linkages Between Informal and Formal Care of the Elderly." *Canadian Journal on Aging/La Revue Canadienne du Vieillissement* 16 (1).

Dhawan, S. (1998). *Caregiving Stress and Acculturation in East Indian Immigrants: Caring for Their Elders.* Ph.D, Kingston, ON: Queen's University.

Dillon, L. (Forthcoming). "Elderly Women in Late Victorian Canada," in B. Hesketh and C. Hackett (eds.), *Canada: Confederation to Present (CD-Rom).* Edmonton: University of Alberta Press.

———— (1998). "Parent-Child Co-Residence Among the Elderly in 1871 Canada and 1880 United States: A Comparative Study," in E.-A. Montigny and A.L. Chambers (eds.), *Family Matters: Papers in Post-Confederation Canadian Family History.* Toronto: Canadian Scholars' Press.

Dorazio-Migliore, M. (1999). *Eldercare in Context: Narrative, Gender, and Ethnicity.* Ph.D, Vancouver: University of British Columbia.

Doyle, V.M. (1989). *Homesharing Matchup Agencies for Seniors: A Literature Review*. Burnaby, BC: Gerontology Research Centre, Simon Fraser University.

Echenberg, H. (1998). *Income Security and Support for Persons with Disabilities: Future Directions*. Ottawa: Canadian Labour Congress.

Eichler, M. (2000). "Contemporary and Historical Diversity in Families: Comment on Turcotte's and Smart's Papers." *Canadian Journal of Family Law* 17 (2).

Esteves, E. (2000). "The New Wageless Worker: Volunteering and Market-Guided Health Care Reform," in D.L. Gustafson (ed.), *Care and Consequences: The Impact of Health Care Reform*. Halifax: Fernwood.

Finch, J. and D. Groves. (1983). *A Labour of Love: Women, Work, and Caring*. London, Boston: Routledge and K. Paul.

Frederick, J.A. and J.E. Fast. (1999). "Eldercare in Canada: Who Does How Much?" *Canadian Social Trends* (Autumn).

Fuller, C. (2002). "The Information Gap: The Impact of Health Care Reform on British Columbia Women," in Pat Armstrong et al., *Exposing Privatization: Women and Health Care Reform in Canada*. Aurora: Garamond Press.

Gignac, M.A.M., E.K. Kelloway and B.H. Gottlieb. (1996). "Impact of Caregiving on Employment: A Mediational Model of Work-Family Conflict." *Canadian Journal on Aging/La Revue Canadienne du Vieillissement* 15 (4).

Guest, D. (1980). *The Emergence of Social Security in Canada*. Vancouver: University of British Columbia Press.

Gurevich, M. (1999). *Privatization in Health Reform from Women's Perspectives: Research, Policy and Responses*. Halifax: Maritime Centre of Excellence for Women's Health.

Gutman, G.M. (1995). *Literature Review: Characteristics, Service Needs and Service Preferences of Younger Adults with Severe Physical Disabilities*. Burnaby, BC: Gerontology Research Centre, Simon Fraser University.

——— (1989). *Survey of Canadian Homesharing Agencies Serving the Elderly*. Burnaby, BC: Gerontology Research Centre, Simon Fraser University.

Gutman, G.M. and N.K. Blackie. (1988). *Housing the Very Old*. Burnaby, BC: Gerontology Research Centre, Simon Fraser University.

Hall, M. and Statistics Canada. (1998). *Caring Canadians, Involved Canadians: Highlights from the 1997 National Survey of Giving, Volunteering and Participating*. Ottawa: Statistics Canada.

Jenson, J. and S. Jacobzone. (2000). *Care Allowances for the Frail Elderly and Their Impact on Women Care-Givers*. Paris, France: Organisation for Economic Co-operation and Development. Directorate for Education Employment Labour and Social Affairs.

Keating, N.C., J. Fast, J. Frederick, et al. (1999). *Eldercare in Canada: Context, Content and Consequences*. Ottawa: Statistics Canada, Housing, Family and Social Statistics Division.

Keefe, J.M. and P. Fancey. (1997). "Financial Compensation on Home Help Services: Examining Differences Among Program Recipients." *Canadian Journal on Aging/La Revue Canadienne du Vieillissement* 16 (2).

King, K.M. and P.M. Koop. (1999). "The Influence of the Cardiac Surgery Patient's Sex and Age on Care-Giving Received." *Social Science and Medicine* 48 (12).

Kobayashi, K.M. (2000). *The Nature of Support from Adult Sansei (Third Generation) Children to Older Nisei (Second Generation) Parents in Japanese Canadian Families*. SEDAP Research Paper No. 18. Hamilton: McMaster University.

Lavoie, J.-P. (1995). "Support Groups for Informal Caregivers Don't Work! Refocus the Groups or the Evaluations?" *Canadian Journal on Aging/La Revue Canadienne du Vieillissement* 14 (3).

Layton, J. (2000). *Homelessness: The Making and Unmaking of a Crisis*. Toronto: Penguin.

Lindsay, C. (1999). "Seniors: A Diverse Group Aging Well." *Canadian Social Trends* (Spring).

MacBride-King, J.L. (1999). *Caring About Caregiving: The Eldercare Responsibilities of Canadian Workers and the Impact on Employers*. Ottawa: The Conference Board of Canada.

Marsh, L. (1975). Special Committee on Social Security, *Report on Social Security for Canada, With a New Introduction by the Author and a Preface by Michael Bliss*. Toronto: University of Toronto Press.

McCann, K. and E. Wadsworth. (1992). "The Role of Informal Carers in Supporting Gay Men Who Have HIV Related Illness." *AIDS Care* 4 (1).

McDaniel, S. and R. Lewis. (1998). "Did They or Didn't They? Intergeneration Supports in Families Past: A Case Study of Brigus, Newfoundland, 1920-1945," in E.-A. Montigny and A.L. Chambers (eds.), *Family Matters: Papers in Post-Confederation Canadian Family History*. Toronto: Canadian Scholars' Press.

McDaniel, S.A. (1997). "Serial Employment and Skinny Government: Reforming Caring and Sharing Among Generations." *Canadian Journal on Aging/La Revue Canadienne du Vieillissement* 16 (3).

McGilly, F. (1991). *An Introduction to Canada's Public Social Services: Understanding Income and Health Programs*. Toronto: McClelland and Stewart.

Meshefedjian, G., J. McCusker, F. Bellavance, et al. (1998). "Factors Associated with Symptoms of Depression Among Informal Caregivers of Demented Elders in the Community." *Gerontologist* 38 (2).

Montigny, E.-A. (2000). "Families, Institutions and the State in Late-Nineteenth-Century Ontario," in E.-A. Montigny and A.L. Chambers (eds.), *Ontario Since Confederation: A Reader*. Toronto: University of Toronto Press.

———— (1997). *Foisted Upon the Government? State Responsibilities, Family Obligations, and the Care of the Dependent Aged in Late Nineteenth-Century Ontario*. Montreal: McGill-Queen's University Press.

Montigny, E.-A. and A.L. Chambers (eds.). (1998). *Family Matters: Papers in Post-Confederation Canadian Family History*. Toronto: Canadian Scholars' Press.

Moore, H. (1997). *Caregiving in Parkinson's: A Qualitative Study of the Perceived Impacts on and Needs of Parkinson's Caregivers*. M.Sc, Kingston, ON: Queen's University.

Morris, M., J. Robinson, J. Simpson, et al. (1999). *The Changing Nature of Home Care and Its Impact on Women's Vulnerability to Poverty*. Ottawa: Status of Women in Canada.

Morrongiello, B. and B. Gottlieb. (2000). "Self-Care Among Adults." *Canadian Journal on Aging/La Revue Canadienne du Vieillissement* 19 (1).

Myles, J. (2000). "The Maturation of Canada's Retirement Income System: Income Levels, Income Inequality and Low Income among Older Persons." *Canadian Journal on Aging/La Revue Canadienne du Vieillissement* 19 (3).

National Forum on Health. (1997). "Values Working Group Synthesis Report" in *Canada Health Action: Building on the Legacy. Synthesis Report and Issues Papers*. Ottawa: Public Works and Government Services.

Neysmith, S. (2000). *Restructuring Caring Labour: Discourse, State Practice, and Everyday Life*. Toronto: Oxford University Press.

Ontario Human Rights Commission. (2000). *Discrimination and Age*. Toronto: Ontario Human Rights Commission.

Ontario Ministry of Community and Social Services. (1991). *Redirection of Long-Term Care and Support Service in Ontario*. Toronto: Queen's Printer for Ontario.

O'Rourke, N., B.E. Havercamp, H. Tuokko, et al. (1996). "Relative Contribution of Subjective Factors to Expressed Burden Among Spousal Caregivers of Suspected Dementia Patients." *Canadian Journal on Aging/La Revue Canadienne du Vieillissement* 15 (4).

Parr, J. (1995). *A Diversity of Women: Ontario, 1945-1980*. Toronto: University of Toronto Press.

———— (1990). *The Gender of Breadwinners: Women, Men, and Change in Two Industrial Towns, 1880-1950*. Toronto: University of Toronto Press.

Penning, M.J. (2000). "Self-, Informal and Formal Care: Partnerships in Community-Based and Residential Long-Term Settings." *Canadian Journal on Aging/La Revue Canadienne du Vieillissement* 19 (Supplement 1).

Porter, J. (1965). *The Vertical Mosaic*. Toronto: University of Toronto Press.

Robb, R., M. Denton, A. Gafni, et al. (1999). "Valuation of Unpaid Help by Seniors in Canada: An Empirical Analysis." *Canadian Journal on Aging/La Revue Canadienne du Vieillissement* 18 (4).

Rosenberg, M.W. and E.G. Moore. (1997). "The Health of Canada's Elderly Population: Current Status and Future Implications." *Canadian Medical Association Journal* 157.

Rosenthal, C.J. and A. Martin-Matthews. (1999). *Families as Care-Providers Versus Care-Managers? Gender and Type of Care in a Sample of Employed Canadians.* SEDAP Research Paper No. 4. Hamilton: McMaster University.

Rosenthal, C.J. and L.O. Stone. (1999). *How Much Help Is Exchanged in Families? Towards an Understanding of Discrepant Research Findings.* SEDAP Research Paper No. 2. Hamilton: McMaster University.

Salvatori, P., M. Tremblay, J. Sandys, et al. (1998). "Aging with an Intellectual Disability: A Review of Canadian Literature." *Canadian Journal on Aging/La Revue Canadienne du Vieillissement* 17 (3).

Sauve, R. (1999). *The Current State of Canadian Family Finances 1999 Report.* Ottawa: The Vanier Institute of the Family,.

Simmons, H.G. (1990). *Unbalanced: Mental Health Policy in Ontario, 1930-1989.* Toronto: Wall and Thompson.

Smart, C. (2000). "Stories of Family Life: Cohabitation, Marriage and Social Change." *Canadian Journal of Family Law* 17 (1).

Snell, J.G. (1996). *The Citizen's Wage: The State and the Elderly in Canada, 1900-1951.* Toronto: University of Toronto Press.

———— (1990). "Filial Responsibility Laws in Canada: An Historical Study." *Canadian Journal on Aging/La Revue Canadienne du Vieillissement* 9 (3).

Spencer, C., M. Ashfield and A. Vanderbijl, (1996). *Abuse and Neglect of Older Adults in Community Settings: An Annotated Bibliography.* Burnaby, BC: Gerontology Research Centre, Simon Fraser University.

Statistics Canada. (1997). "Who Cares? Caregiving in the 1990's." *The Daily.*

———— (2000). *Women in Canada.* Ottawa: Ministry of Industry.

Stewart, M. (2000). *Chronic Conditions and Caregiving in Canada: Social Support Strategies.* Toronto: University of Toronto Press.

Struthers, J. (1994). *The Limits of Affluence: Welfare in Ontario, 1920-1970.* Toronto: University of Toronto Press.

Taylor, D. (Forthcoming). "Making Care Visible: Exploring the Healthwork of People Living with HIVAIDS in Ontario."

Taylor, M. (1978). *Health Insurance and Canadian Public Policy.* Kingston: McGill-Queen's University Press.

The Roeher Institute, (2001). *Personal Relationships of Support between Adults: The Case of Disability.* Toronto: The Roeher Institute.

The Vanier Institute of the Family. (n.d.) *The Family, From the Kitchen Table to the Boardroom Table: A Digest.* Ottawa: The Vanier Institute of the Family.

Townson, M. and Canadian Advisory Council on the Status of Women. (1995). *Women's Financial Futures: Mid-Life Prospects for a Secure Retirement.* Ottawa: Canadian Advisory Council on the Status of Women.

Trottier, H., L. Martel, C. Houle, et al. (2000). "Living at Home or in an Institution: What Makes the Difference for Seniors?" *Health Reports* 11 (4).

Ward-Griffin, C. (1998). *Negotiating the Boundaries of Eldercare: The Relationship Between Nurses and Family Caregivers.* Ph.D, Toronto: University of Toronto, Dept. of Public Health Sciences.

Ward-Griffin, C. and P. McKeever. (2000). "Relationships Between Nurses and Family Caregivers: Partners in Care?" *Advances in Nursing Science* 22 (3).

Wilkins, K. and M.P. Beaudet. (2000). "Changes in Social Support in Relation to Seniors' Use of Home Care." *Health Reports* 3 11 (4).

Willson, K. and J. Howard. (2002). "Missing Links: The Effects of Health Care Privatization on Women in Manitoba and Saskatchewan," in Pat Armstrong et al., *Exposing Privatization: Women and Health Care Reform in Canada.* Aurora: Garamond Press.

Wolfson, C., R. Handfield-Jones, K.C. Glass, et al. (1993). "Adult Children's Perceptions of Their Responsibility to Provide Care for Dependent Elderly Parents." *Gerontologist* 33 (3).

Woolley, F. (1998). *Work and Household Transactions: An Economist's View.* Ottawa: Canadian Policy Research Networks Inc.

Yalnizyan, A. (1998). *The Growing Gap: A Report on Growing Inequality Between the Rich and the Poor in Canada.* Toronto: Centre for Social Justice.

Designing Home and Community Care For the Future: Who Needs to Care?[1]

Nancy Guberman

Before answering the question posed in the second part of the title (that is, "Who Needs to Care?") I would like to look at the first half: "Designing Home and Community Care." Examining the concepts of home and community care will ultimately lead me to my answer to the question of who needs to care.

As presented in the title, the terms "home and community care" could suggest that we are talking about two realities, or at least two locations: care in the home and care in the community. But, in fact, in current policy, practice and the lived experience of most people, these two realities are too often collapsed into one reality, and that reality is home care.

Indeed, more often than not, when we talk about community care we are talking about care in the home, supplemented occasionally by day centres. And when we talk about care in the home, more often than not we are talking about care provided mainly by family and friends, supplemented by some homemaking, personal care or nursing support and perhaps Meals-on-Wheels or volunteer transportation services. And among family and friends we are most often talking about women. So, again, more often than not, what is called community care is in fact care by women in the family with little or no support from the community. Today, most people with disabilities and chronic health problems are being cared for in the home, not in the community, and they are being cared for mainly by close female relatives not by the community. For example, in Quebec over 81.2 percent of all people with disabilities are living in private homes (Statistics Canada 1996). Of these, approximately half need help to accomplish their daily activities (Institut de la statistique du Québec 1998) and 80 percent of this help is offered by family members (Garant and Bolduc 1990; Stone et al. 1987).

THE SHIFT TO COMMUNITY CARE

It is important to situate this reality within the context of the restructuring of the state. Since the 1980s the Canadian state,[2] like the rest of the Western world, has been faced with a number of "crises," including a financial crisis and a crisis as to the legitimacy of its intervention in the social realm and, in particular, into family life. The welfare state has been criticized for its bureaucratic and technocratic intervention, as well as for being the source of excessive demands for equality that have led to the breakup of the family (Eisenstein 1984; Guberman 1987). The political philosophy of the welfare state has given way to a recentring of state social intervention around "social protection" rather than universal insurance-type programs (Lesemann 1988; Lesemann and Lamoureux 1987; Walker 1987; Webb and Wistow 1987). State intentions are clear: reduce the costs of its services, deinstitutionalize its ways of assuring care and transfer and share its responsibilities with other stakeholders, including the private sector. In terms of long-term care policy, this has led various provincial governments to announce clearly that the state must no longer intervene in such a way as to substitute for other stakeholders who can and should be providing care, notably family members (Quebec 1985, Ontario 1986).[3]

This shift to an ideology of shared responsibility for care has been accompanied by drastic cutbacks in health and social service budgets, both in terms of federal transfer payments and within provincial budgets. The new focus on care outside the hospital and the residential institution is seen as politically legitimate, more cost-effective, and also as providing better patient care in more appropriate settings based on studies of the determinants of health (Armstrong et al. 1994).

The common assumption is that the social and emotional support that people need for good health can best be received in their own homes. As well, the shift to community care answers certain administrative needs, such as reducing hospital waiting lists and meeting the challenges of changing demography, seen by governments as the "grey menace."

However, it has been clearly documented that community care is often a euphemism for unpaid family care (Finch and Groves 1983). It is estimated that families have always assumed the lion's share of care to dependent members of society, with figures ranging from 75 percent to 90 percent of care being provided by family members and friends (Brody 1990; Chappell et al. 1986; Garant and Bolduc 1990). Today, social policies and programs addressing disabled and ill persons are frequently predicated on the assumption that the family is now the preferred locus and provider of care. Services are no longer offered as an entitlement, but rather as a backup to family incapacity to assure care. The shift to "community" care has been, at least in part, a shift from statutory to voluntary, from formal to informal and from paid to unpaid care.

Care in the Home as the Popular Choice

But, we are often told, people want to be cared for in their homes. It is their first choice. To better understand this phenomenon, we must look at how the choices for long-term care are represented. The reduction of community care to care in the home finds some of its ideological underpinnings in the current dichotomous vision of care as being either home care or institutional care. They are basically the only two options currently on offer and only one of those options, that is, care in the home, is considered really viable.

As they exist today, care in the home or care in an alternative setting are presented almost dichotomously as good and bad.

INSTITUTIONS	FAMILIES
cold, unfeeling	warmth, emotional bonds
professionals	lay
wages	love
technical interventions	spontaneous/simple
lack of freedom	freedom
regimentation	absence of schedules

Given these images, the choice is simple. Institutionalization is seen as a last resort by most people with disabilities or health problems that require home care, and also most caregivers. It is so socially depreciated as an option that it is more like a non-choice. Add to the equation the current severely restricted access to institutional beds and the home appears to be the best and only option. Therefore, despite the numerous documented difficulties of caring and being cared for at home, this appears to be the only real choice available.

However, there are many indications that people might choose different solutions if only they had different options available to them. First, it is clear that people with sufficient means generally buy the services and hire the people required to meet their needs as they grow frailer or develop disabilities, rather than choosing to be cared for by family and friends. Family members and friends continue to offer emotional and social support but do not do most of the hands-on activities required unless they and the person with disabilities freely choose this option. It is considered acceptable, and often desirable, for a wealthy senior to move into a seniors' village or private residence with adapted facilities and meal, laundry, housekeeping and on-site medical services. However, the appeal of these options is the fact that people maintain control over their own lives – they have their own private spaces and they have options available to them with regard to services and programs.

Second, the first choice of most people with disabilities is not to be dependent on or a burden to their families. Research shows that they want to maintain intimacy at a distance (Shanas 1979). Daatland (1990:10-11 in Neysmith 1991) describing the Norwegian situation, explains:

> The contrast between what responsibility an adult child will accept for old parents, and the responsibility the elderly are willing to impose on their own children, may go to the core of the issue. Parents are afraid of

overloading their children, and use alternatives when they have a reasonably good choice. Like all persons, young and old alike, they find it easier to give than to receive; easier to be the independent provider than the dependent receiver. One-sided dependency has probably never been productive for good family relations.

Younger persons with physical, mental or intellectual disabilities, those in their twenties, thirties or forties, generally want a chance to strike out on their own. They feel it is not normal to still be living with, or be dependent on, their parents.

And yet, based on current practices where, in the face of non-choice, people with disabilities are being cared for at home by family and friends for as long as possible, we are told by policy-makers that family care is the most natural and moral option, and the choice of most Canadians.

I propose that home care as it exists today is neither the most natural nor the most moral option and I am far from sure that it is indeed the first choice of most Canadians. I believe we have to shift paradigms and start asking questions: How can we as a society provide people needing support or care with options that offer them as much independence, choice and autonomy as possible given their individual situations; options that enable them to participate to the fullest extent possible as active, integrated citizens, while offering the safety, security and support they need? As one key informant to a recent policy paper questioned: "Can we write a long-term care policy without once mentioning the word 'family'?" (Guberman 1999).

Before examining some of the options concerning a new model of community care, it is important to analyze what I believe are some major shortcomings in current policy choices and their underlying premises.

CURRENT POLICY AND ITS ASSUMPTIONS

In direct contradiction to the appeal for a non-family-based paradigm of long-term care, it would appear that the federal and provincial governments have, to date, opted for a policy approach wherein families are the cornerstone of the care package and services are given to supplement but never substitute for family care. Any direct services to caregivers to support them in their tasks or to help them cope with any untoward consequences of caregiving are intended to shore them up so that they may continue, never to give them any option of scaling back or stopping care. This approach reinforces rather than attenuates the idea of family responsibility. It is in no way offered as a strategy for sharing the care and yet this orientation is masked behind a discourse of developing a partnership between families and the state.

The decision to rely heavily on the family as the cornerstone of long-term care, as developed above, appears to be the result of perceived budgetary and other resource constraints (Keating et al. 1997). Indeed, policy debates concerning support to caregivers are most often framed in terms of the need to reduce or control expenditures and achieve a balance between incentives and disincentives to family care (Osterbusch et al. 1987). There seems to be much concern that the provision of services will lead to family abdication, despite the reality that caregivers are difficult to recruit for most programs which are aimed at them and that families tend to delay their requests for service until the situation has become overwhelming. Also, research has shown that there is no hard evidence that families decrease their involvement and substitute formal care for their own contribution when such care is available, although they may modify the nature of their activities (Brody 1995; Chappell 1992; Kane and Penrod 1995).

What governments do not seem to consider is the capacity of families and women to assume the role that the state has scripted for them. Is it possible to reconcile the aim of revitalizing family responsibility for disabled members with the realities of families as we enter the third millennium? Does this approach not overestimate families' and women's capacities and competencies? Given the nature and level of disabilities of people being maintained at home and their care requirements, given the economic necessity for all adults in the family to be in the labour force, given the breakdown of traditional family structures and the complexity of new family relationships, do families have the concrete conditions to assure quality care to disabled kin without undue negative consequences to the caregiver, and possibly the care recipient, which may in the long run be more costly to the state?

Underlying policy that aims at shoring up families as the cornerstone of long-term care are assumptions about "the family." The monolithic term "the family," which is often used in policy and programs, assumes that there is only one legitimate family form and that this family includes at least one member available in the home to assume the responsibilities for care that the state wants to transfer. In other words, policy tends to uphold an idealized view of the traditional family and promotes women's proper role as being in the home to care for other family members. References to "the family," or even to "caregivers," in policy and programs also hide the gendered nature of family caregiving.

Romanticizing Family Care

A policy approach based on the centrality of family caregiving is also based on assumptions about the harmony and security of family life. The ideology of family care presumes that uncompensated care is kinder, more sensitive, more attuned to individual needs. Moore (1991) for example, advances that the primary group is more effective than formal services because caring work is unpredictable and cannot be easily subdivided. Litvak (1985) has theorized about which social tasks are best performed by the formal sector and which are best left to kin and the informal sector, and concludes that formal organizations can never provide the quality of care that families provide given the latter's resiliency, flexibility and emotional commitment.

And yet, care within the family is not necessarily loving, adapted or in the best interests of persons with disabilities. Even if some families are organized on the basis of affection and mutual help, we cannot forget that many families are also the site of interpersonal and intergenerational conflicts, abuse and violence. Caregiving to dependent family members can lead to the fracturing of family ties and bitter conflicts among family members (Abel 1987; Guberman et al. 1991).

The premise that advances the family as the ideal location for care ignores the reality of the solitude and the unhappiness of many people who are isolated in their families. Agnès Pitrou (1992) asks if the fact that more and more people claim that they turn first and foremost to their family for aid is an indicator of the value they place on this institution or if it is not, on the contrary, an indicator of the poverty of their social networks and the problems of accessibility to collective resources. The need to fall back on the family could be taken as much as a sign of failure and lack of choice as a fact that should be glorified. Research has demonstrated that the more financial and personal resources you have, the less likely you are to be limited to mutual aid within your family and the more likely you are to benefit from collective services.

Furthermore, policy that assumes that emotional attachments can only exist in kin reationships overlooks the fact that personal benefits can be associated with formal service delivery (Hooyman and Gonyea 1995). Qureshi and Walker (1989) found that some people experience the receipt of formal services as an expression of caring on the part of their relatives, not as a sign of abdication. It is clear too that many formal service providers develop personal affective relations with those to whom they provide care. History offers us many examples where paid care and personalized affection exist in combination, including experiences with nannies, domestic workers and the many women in the underground economy who are hired to care for children and adults with disabilities (Waerness 1987).

A policy approach that is aimed at reinforcing family care also ignores the concrete conditions of Canadian families as we move into the twenty-first century. Most adults in families are in the workforce or on welfare workfare and have little availability for providing care. More and more families are seeing their incomes approaching or falling below the poverty level. Given the skyrocketing costs of housing in major urban centres, many families are moving to smaller housing units. A record number of people are living alone or in non-traditional family forms (e.g., long-distance relationships, gay couples, reconstituted families) which means that their availability for providing care may be more limited or challenging. This approach also ignores the fact that it is not the family but generally one woman in the family, often a woman who is aging herself and with her own health problems, who assumes the care. Do these families, these women, have the conditions to offer quality care? And what of the numerous documented impacts of this policy approach on women as caregivers?

Putting Into Question Norms of Universality and Equity
Another question raised by the government transfer of care to women in the home concerns the effect of decentralizing care into as many sub-units as there are families who are assuming this care. This will lead to the quality and quantity of care, services and resources which a person is entitled to being

dependent on the competencies, availability and resourcefulness of their family member. Families cannot offer more than what they dispose of in terms of security, hygiene and other material conditions and, considering that these conditions are as variable as there are variations in family situations, the increased centrality of families in the organization of care runs the risk of increasing social inequalities.

As Anne Bullock (1990:75) comments: "The notion of a community that relies on the 'family' for its existence is a contradiction. Community implies egalitarian social organization that benefits all of its members. Family implies a privatized, hierarchical and gendered work organization that does not equally benefit its members and also foments the differences among families who are thought to comprise 'the community'."

A family approach also ignores the reality of the growing number of single older people. Single and divorced elderly men are a particularly vulnerable group who risk having no family members willing to assure their care.

Women's "Choice" to Care

Research reveals that it is erroneous to affirm that women choose to care for sick and elderly relatives or that for all women their only, or even principal, motive for assuming caregiving is love and self-sacrifice. Although there may be very strong emotional ties between caregiver and care receiver, it is also true that caregiving relations are structured in a coercive way given the absence of real choice and true alternatives in a society based on the sexual division of labour (Guberman et al. 1991, 1992; Neysmith 1991). Thurer (1983) notes that women have unavoidably filled the vacuum left by insufficient community services as an extension of their culturally appointed nurturing role. Guberman et al. (1992) found that three of the six primary factors that appear to be determinants of a woman's decision to provide care represent external or structural constraints: the inadequacy of institutional and community resources, the imposition of the decision by the dependent person and women's economic dependency.

Feminist analysts (Abel 1991; Aronson 1991; Baines et al. 1991; Dalley 1988; Finch and Groves 1983; Estes et al. 1993; Guberman et al. 1992 ; Hooyman and Gonyea 1995) thus point to the necessity to break down the dichotomies of public versus private and impersonal public care versus loving home care and challenge the gendered division of labour in all its forms.

Current policy based on family ideology must be criticized because it is based on erroneous premises and is harmful to women's well-being as both caregivers and persons with disabilities. As caregivers, women often do not have the material and moral conditions to take on the responsibilities that the state is attempting to transfer to them. Moreover, state policy ignores the well-documented negative consequences that this situation has for a majority of caregivers (Biegel et al. 1991; Cranswick 1997; Fast et al. 1999; Gottlieb et al. 1994; Strawbridge and Wallhagen 1991; Zarit 1991). As well, despite different attempts to develop interventions to reduce these consequences, the varied fragmented measures and programs that do exist have not been shown to have any major impact on caregiver well-being (American Medical Association 1993; Armstrong et al. 1994; Flint 1995; Knight et al. 1993; Hooyman and Gonyea 1995; Zarit et al. 1998). Finally, recent studies question the quality and appropriateness of care when it is assumed by lay people and the impact this has on people with disabilities (Arras and Dubler 1995; Daniels 1995; Gagnon et al. 2001; Kane 1995). These elements clearly call for a change of paradigm.

How can we then design community care that takes into account these issues while still responding to the needs of people with disabilities?

WHAT WOULD GENUINE COMMUNITY CARE LOOK LIKE?

This section will present what has been called a social model of community care. It is more of a framework than a blueprint for policy-makers and program designers – that is, it provides the framework for community care policies and programs, but it has to be fleshed out and adapted by the people most concerned (people with disabilities, caregivers, feminists and professionals). It is not an original model – it takes much inspiration from work by Sheila Neysmith and her collabourators in Canada and Nancy Hooyman and Judith Gonyea in the United States.

This model conflicts with current dominant assumptions about the role and responsibilities of families and government for providing care for people with disabilities. It also may appear unrealistic given the prevailing economic and political climate. But beyond economic concerns, issues of justice and equity should push us in this direction.

Central Principle: Care Needs Are Seen as a Social Issue and a Social Responsibility

A social model of community care would start from the premise that caregiving to disabled or ill members of society is a social responsibility. It recognizes care as a social problem and caregiving as true work. It fosters social messages and a social organization which does not oblige families to be the main providers of instrumental and emotional help to dependent family members. Empowerment and choice are central to this model, as is the development of a partnership between all concerned stakeholders: people with disabilities, family caregivers, the public sector, the private sector, the voluntary sector and the community, a partnership orchestrated by the state and organized around a strong public presence. Social responsibility implies that the public sector remains at the centre of service organization, that public services are available to people who need them as an entitlement right of citizenship. Those who choose to assume caregiving would not be penalized by unresponsive labour practices; nor would they incur financial and career losses. Within the partnership, a clearly defined role for the private sector would need to be developed.

As Dumont-Lemasson (1994) suggests, public home care services should be the strategic link and the cornerstone of aging policy. I would add that this applies to all policy concerning disabled persons. I would also broaden the range of Dumont-Lemasson's statement to include not only health and social services, but also housing, employment, recreation, urban development services, etc. Dumont-Lemasson argues that public home care services, at least as they exist in Quebec, offer several advantages over the private for-profit and voluntary sectors. They have only a social finality,[4] they can orient clients within the entire health and social service system and within other government systems, they offer the quality of trained and supervised personnel, a multidisciplinary approach, the protection of vulnerable individuals and accountability. Many of these characteristics are also true of the other public services cited.

To promote empowerment and genuine choice, a social model must assure that the measures, programs and services offered by the public sector and other stakeholders are characterized by flexibility, adaptability, variety, continuity, coordination and the organized input of people with disabilities and caregivers. Another aspect of the model is that it promotes a global and holistic vision of care.

With this approach, responsibility for caregiving does not rest primarily on families and caregivers. The care needs of people with disabilities are considered a social issue requiring a collective solution. They cannot be reduced to a family or individual responsibility.

ORIENTATIONS OF A SOCIAL MODEL OF CARE

Genuine Choice to Assume Caregiving

Choices in terms of caregiving arrangements are always dependent on one's social conditions, economic status, knowledge of available resources, capacity to analyze the costs/benefits of different options and capacity to make a decision. To truly have the possibility of choice, there has to be a balance between a person's individual values, conditions, capacities and skill at making choices, and concrete viable options from which to choose. These options must be of equal social value to be real choices. For example, as indicated earlier in this chapter, one can now choose between family care and institutionalization but the latter is so socially depreciated as an option that it is almost a non-choice. In this situation, family care is a non-choice because there are not viable, socially acceptable alternatives. It is a non-choice because choice has been dichotomized as one between warm, loving, caring families and cold, bureaucratic uncaring institutions. But just as reality is more complex than that, so too do solutions have to be more complex than that.

Choice and the quality of care are dependent upon the existence of an array of support resources in sufficient quantity (England et al. 1990) including sufficient residential alternatives when the choice is not to be cared for at home (McConnell and Riggs 1994). By residential alternatives I am not referring to long-term care facilities as we know them today, but rather to a variety of small-scale residences with services integrated into the community: group homes, sheltered housing, supervised apartments, satellite homes around long-term care facilities, etc.

When people with disabilities and a family member or friend do agree to caregiving at home, they must be supported by a comprehensive range of accessible, integrated and culturally appropriate services (Ansello and Roberto 1993). Given the diversity of caregivers and caregiving situations, the services, measures and supports must be wide-ranging and varied.

The essential core of a model of social community care is the organization of a continuum of community-based services, financed mainly by the state, which are accessible, adapted and flexible with a single point of entry and a single assessment. Within this organization, we would find third-party advocates whose role is to help caregivers and care recipients negotiate through the system and to defend their rights.

Current home care services must be substantially increased, particularly housekeeping and psychosocial services, and an array of new innovative services should be added aimed at maximizing the autonomy and assuring the highest possible level of integration of people with disabilities into all aspects of society.

Care as a Right of Citizenship

When caring is seen as a social responsibility, access to services becomes a right of citizenship (Neysmith 1991). Each individual is entitled to these services regardless of his or her family situation and a minimum floor of adequate support should be assured to all disabled individuals (Kane and Penrod 1995). This means guaranteeing sufficient funding of community-based services. Universal access to a guaranteed minimum of services assures equity among people and will work against the development of a two-tiered system wherein only those with sufficient financial resources can access a variety of supports in the for-profit sector. It also counters the current situation where the quality and quantity of care that a person receives are mainly determined by the competency, availability, resourcefulness and circumstances of the individual's family. It may also prevent the fracturing of family ties and bitter conflicts among family members that are currently the outcome of caregiving in some families.

Building Communities for the Integration of People With Disabilities

Building community for the genuine integration of people with disabilities implies developing a partnership between all concerned stakeholders: people with disabilities, caregivers, the private not-for-profit, the private for-profit sector, the voluntary sector and the community, a partnership orchestrated by the state. The various stakeholders are mobilized around their specific areas of expertise. Building community means designing geographically and architecturally accessible neighbourhoods and towns, including efficient adapted transportation, particularly in rural communities, and adapted recreation facilities for example. It can also mean undertaking media campaigns to change attitudes and behaviours towards the disabled, the ill and the elderly, or stronger incentives to integrate people with disabilities into the workforce.

Promotion of Global Vision of Health, Prevention and Management of Disease

Another aspect of the model, as stated by Hooyman and Gonyea, is that it promotes "a redefinition of health that integrates social and health services, physical and mental health care, and prevention as well as treatment" (1995:327). It also takes into account the reality that caregiving is often long-term. Furthermore, this model is not disease-specific and does not dichotomize between chronic and acute care.

People who are frail or suffer from acute illness, chronic illness, mental illness or mental handicaps are heterogeneous in terms of the course of their illness or disability, their care needs and their degree of dependency. However, they face many common issues in terms of dominant health models, interface with formal services and the impact of public policy geared towards community care. As well, their family caregivers face many common issues including the consequences of caregiving on their lives and the lack of explicit consideration of their situation in policy and programs. Indeed, caregivers may have more commonalities across diseases than is generally believed and differences may be more closely linked to onset, disease course, likely outcome and level of incapacity. Interventions guided by disease could give way to interventions guided by the source of caregiver stress or the circumstances of the person with disabilities and their caregiver. This could lead to merged funding streams to meet the needs of a cross-section of persons with incapacities and caregivers, and to cross-disease advocacy groups of caregivers (Ansello and Roberto 1993; Hooyman and Gonyea 1995).

Another aspect of a more global vision of health would put more emphasis on promoting functional autonomy. Researchers and practitioners have advanced a number of strategies for minimizing the impact of functional limitations on people's daily lives (Garant and Bolduc 1990). First among these is increased access to rehabilitation programs for people with disabilities without prejudice as to their age, place of residency or disability. While rehabilitation is not a panacea, it can reduce incapacities or develop compensatory skills. Adapting houses and communities to answer the practical needs of the disabled – and, in fact, any actions that could reduce the difficulties inherent in daily activities – should be promoted, as should access to technical aids, prostheses and other equipment that enables people with disabilities to compensate for certain functional deficits due to their condition. To this, Estes et al. (1993) add the need to provide explicit training to people with disabilities so they can develop skills to cope with daily stresses.

Input From People With Disabilities and Caregivers

Input from people with disabilities and caregivers at all levels of the health care system, from conception to evaluation, is a major aspect of this model. Their involvement would ensure that their situations are truly recognized, appreciated and taken into consideration in all decisions. People with disabilities and caregivers alike should not only participate fully, they should include delegation from consumer advocacy groups so that representatives truly represent a constituency. The capacity of these delegates to represent their group and participate in decisions concerning policy, planning and implementation will be enhanced by the existence of consumer rights groups working from an empowerment approach.

This approach is aimed at supporting people as they take control over their lives and, in the case of caregivers, as they gain control over the choices they must make in their lives. Gutiérrez's (1990) definition of empowerment is very appropriate for caregivers and includes maximizing a sense of personal control over one's decisions combined with the ability to affect the behaviour of others, a focus on enhancing existing strengths in individuals and communities, a goal of establishing equity in the distribution of resources and a structural rather than individual or victim-blaming form of analysis for understanding problems. Advocacy groups work to develop a collective consciousness and a collective identity, thus reducing self-blame. Their interventions look to the structural origins of problems so that caregivers can focus on changing the source of the problem rather than only changing themselves. These groups must be assured of stable, long-term funding to fulfill this mandate.

For caregivers to have control over their choices they must make informed decisions. This requires education about their options. Since reaching caregivers is often very difficult, Hooyman and Gonyea suggest that educational sessions about caregiving and long-term care be integrated into natural settings such as Employee Assistance Programs, community centres and adult education classes. In this way they would have the added benefit of reaching potential caregivers and other family members, and acting as a preventive measure.

Would care in the home continue to be the preferred choice of people with disabilities and family and friends if genuine community care were available? After all, caring by families and friends does not end because a person is in some form of alternative residential setting. Keating (1998) found that 30 percent of direct services of institutionalized older people were being provided by family members. While this is surely a reflection of the under-funding and lack of resources in today's institutions it is also a sign of family involvement with kin no matter where they are housed.

WHO SHOULD CARE?

I now come to the second half of the question posed at the outset. Who needs to care? Well, obviously, many of us already do care. We know that family and friends provide between 80 percent and 90 percent of all care to people with disabilities at home and that over two-thirds of these caregivers are women. Studies consistently document that women form between two-thirds and three-quarters of all caregivers (Garant and Bolduc 1990; Statistics Canada 1996; Stone et al. 1987). According to Statistics Canada, this means that at any one time 14 percent of all Canadian women over fifteen years of age were caregivers (Statistics Canada 1996). Women already care in their paid roles as homemakers, nurses, social workers, rehab personnel, etc., but we are currently caring as if care were an individual or family affair.

I, therefore, believe we have to switch our thinking and start asking how we can best promote independent living and quality of care for people with disabilities. How can we make care a social issue?

I also believe we have to start thinking about equity and justice for all people with disabilities and about gender equity and justice for women who care as paid and unpaid caregivers.

But most of all, I believe our governments, politicians and policy-makers need to care. Despite short-term economic setbacks we are a rich society. We have the means to offer genuine social community care. We have always believed in free and universal health care, in equity and social justice. To design home and community care which reflect these values, we must work to protect, reaffirm and reinforce them and make the type of model that I am proposing a political priority. Then we will all care.

Notes

1. Parts of this chapter are a modified version of sections of Guberman, N. (1999). Caregivers and Caregiving: New Trends and their Implications for Policy. Report prepared for Health Canada, document miméo.

2. I am employing the term Canadian state to refer to federal, provincial and territorial governments.

3. "Professional services should be used to enhance and supplement, not replace, family support services." (Ontario Ministry of Community and Social Services, 1988:8) "The manifest implication of the state and the means it has privileged (institutional care) contribute to individuals and groups becoming dependent upon state services. The resulting demobilization discourages the maximal use of the potential provided by individual, family and community energies." (Ministère des affaires sociales 1985:28) "The services available to elderly persons must be better adapted to their needs and their aspirations; however, these cannot replace the contribution of the elderly persons themselves or that of their milieu." (57).

4. As part of non-profit para-public agencies, Quebec home care services receive statutory, albeit insufficient, annual funding from the government. Compared to the for-profit sector, they have in their mission only social goals and in contrast to non-profits in the rest of Canada, they do not have to bid for contracts. They also are responsible for both the assessment of need and the service delivery to meet these needs.

References

Abel, E.K. (1987). *Love is Not enough: Family Care of the Frail Elderly.* Washington, D.C.: American Public Health Association.

———— (1991). *Who Cares for the Elderly?* Philadelphia: Temple University Press.

American Medical Association, Council on Scientific Affairs. (1993). "Physicians and Family Caregivers." *Journal of the American Medical Association,* 269(10), 1282-1284.

Ansello, E.F. and K.A. Roberto. (1993). "Empowering Elderly Caregivers: Practice, Research and Policy Directions" in K.A. Roberto (ed.), *The Elderly Caregiver: Caring for Adults With Developmental Disabilities.* Newbury Park, CA: Sage.

Armstrong, P., H. Armstrong, J. Choinière, G. Feldberg and J. White. (1994). *Take Care: Warning Signals for Canada's Health System.* Toronto: Garamond Press.

Aronson, J. (1991). "Dutiful Daughters and Undemanding Mothers: Contrasting Images of Giving and Receiving Care in Middle and Later Life," p. 138-168 in C. Baines, P. Evans and S. Neysmith (eds.), *Women's Caring: Feminist Perspectives on Social Welfare.* Toronto: McClelland and Stewart.

Arras, J.D. and N.N. Dubler. (1995). "Ethical and Social Implications of High-Tech Home Care," p. 15-28 in J.D. Arras, W.H. Porterfield and L.O. Porterfield (eds.), *Bringing the Hospital Home: Ethical and Social Implications of High-tech Home Care.* Baltimore: The Johns Hopkins University Press.

Baines, C., P. Evans and S. Neysmith. (1991). *Women's Caring: Feminist Perspectives on Social Welfare.* Toronto: McClelland and Stewart.

Biegel, D., E. Sales and R. Schulz. (1991). *Family Caregiving in Chronic Illness.* Newbury Park, CA: Sage.

Brody, E.M. (1990). *Women in the Middle: Their Parent-care Years.* New York: Springer Pub. Co.

———— (1995). "Prospects for Family Caregiving" in R.A. Kane and J.D. Penrod (eds.), *Family Caregiving in an Aging Society.* Thousand Oaks, CA: Sage Publications.

Bullock, A. (1990). "Community Care: Ideology and Lived Experience" in R. Ng, G. Walker and J. Muller (eds.), *Community Organization and the Canadian State.* Toronto: Garamond Press.

Chappell, N.L. (1992). *Social Support and Aging.* Toronto: Butterworths.

Chappell, N.L., L.A. Strain and A.A. Blanford. (1986). *Aging and Health Care: A Social Perspective.* Toronto: Holt, Rinehart and Winston.

Côté, D. et al. (1998). *Qui donnera les soins?: Les incidences du virage ambulatoire et des mesures d'économie sociale sur les femmes du Québec.* Ottawa: Condition féminine Canada.

Cranswick, K. (1997). "Canada's Caregivers." *Canadian Social Trends,* 47, 2-6.

Daatland, S. (1994). "Recent Trends and Future Prospects for the Elderly in Scandinavia." *Journal of Aging & Social Policy,* 6(1-2):181-197.

Dalley, G. (1988). *Ideologies of Caring: Rethinking Community and Collectivism.* London: Macmillan.

Daniels, N (1995). "Justice and Access to High-Tech Home Care," p. 197-219 in J.D. Arras, W.H. Porterfield and L.O. Porterfield (eds.), *Bringing the Hospital Home: Ethical and Social Implications of High-Tech Home Care.* Baltimore: The Johns Hopkins University Press.

Dumont-Lemasson, M. (1994). "Des services de soutien à domicile fragiles pour une clientèle vulnerable." *Service Social,* 43(1), 47-65.

Eisenstein, Z. (1984). *Feminism and Sexual Equality: Crisis in Liberal America.* New York: Monthly Review Press.

England, S.E. (1990). "Family Leave and Gender Justice." *Affilia: Journal of Women and Social Work,* 5, 8-15.

England, S.E., S.M. Keigher, B. Miller and N.C. Linsk. (1990). "Community Care Policies" in M. Minkler and C. Estes (eds.), *Critical Perspectives on Aging: The Political and Moral Economy of Growing Old.* Amityville, N.Y.: Baywood.

Estes, C., J. Swan and Associates. (1993). *The Long-term Care Crisis.* Newbury Park, CA: Sage.

Fast. J.E., D.L. Williamson and N.C. Keating. (1999). "The Hidden Costs of Informal Elder Care." *Journal of Family and Economic Issues,* 20(3):301-326.

Finch, J. and D. Groves. (1983). *A Labour of Love: Women, Work and Caring.* London: Routledge and Kegan Paul.

Flint, A.J. (1995). "Effects of Respite Care on Patients With Dementia and Their Caregivers." *International Psychogeriatrics*, 7(4), 505-517.

Gagnon, E. (2001). *Les impacts du virage ambulatoire: responsabilités et encadrement dans la dispensation des soins à domicile.* Québec, Direction de la santé publique et régie régionale de la santé et des services sociaux de Québec.

Gagnon, E., N. Guberman et al. (2001). *Les impacts du virage ambulatoire: responsabilités et encadrement dans la dispensation des soins à domicile. Québec: Direction de la santé publique et régie régionale de la santé et des services sociaux de Québec.*

Garant, L. and M. Bolduc. (1990). *L'Aide par les proches: Mythes et réalités.* Québec. Direction de l'évaluation, ministère de la Santé et des Services sociaux. Québec: Les Publications du Québec.

Gottlieb, B.H., E.K. Kelloway and M. Fraboni. (1994). "Aspects of Eldercare That Place Employees at Risk." *The Gerontologist*, 34(6), 815-821.

Guberman, N. (1987). "Discours de responsabilisation des familles et retrait de l'État-providence" in R. Dandurand (ed.), *Couples et parents des années quatre-vingt. Un aperçu de nouvelles tendances.* Questions de culture, no. 13. Québec: IQRC.

Guberman, N. (1999). *Caregivers and Caregiving: New Trends and Their Implications for Policy.* Report prepared for Health Canada, document mimeo.

Guberman, N., P. Maheu and C. Maillé. (1991). *Et si l'amour ne suffisait pas?: Femmes, familles et adultes dépendants.* Montréal: Les éditions du Remue-ménage.

——— (1992). "Women as Family Caregivers: Why do They Care?" *The Gerontologist*, 32(5), 607-617.

Gutiérrez, L. (1990). "Working With Women of Color: An Empowerment Perspective." *Social Work.* 35(2), 192-197.

Hooyman, N. and J. Gonyea. (1995). *Feminist Perspectives on Family Care: Policies for Gender Justice.* Thousand Oaks, CA: Sage Publications.

Institut de la statistique du Québec. (1998). *Enquête québécoise sur les limitations d'activitiés, 1998.* Quebec: Gouvernement du Québec (2001).

Kane, R.A. (1995). "High-tech Home Care in Context: Organizations, Quality and Ethical Ramifications," p. 197-219 in J.D. Arras, W.H. Porterfield and L.O. Porterfield (eds), *Bringing the Hospital Home: Ethical and Social Implications of High-tech Home Care.* Baltimore: The Johns Hopkins University Press.

Kane, R.A. and J.D. Penrod. (1995). "Toward a Caregiving Policy for the Aging Family," p.140-170 in R.A. Kane and J.D. Penrod (eds.), *Family Caregiving in an Aging Society: Policy Perspectives.* Thousand Oaks, CA: Sage Publications Inc.

Keating, N.C. (1998). *Evaluating Programs of Innovative Continuing Care: Final Report.* Edmonton: University of Alberta Press.

Keating, N.C., J.E. Fast, I.A Connidis, M. Penning and J. Keefe. (1997). "Bridging Policy and Research in Eldercare." *Canadian Journal on Aging.* Special Issue, 22-41.

Knight, B.G., S.M. Lutzky and F. Macofsky-Urban. (1993). "A Meta-analytic Review of Interventions for Caregiver Distress: Recommendations for Future Research. *The Gerontologist*, 33(2), 240-248.

Lesemann, F. (1988). *La politique sociale américaine.* Paris: Syros.

Lesemann, F. and J. Lamoureux. (1987). *Le rôle et le devenir de l'État-providence.* Commission d'enquête sur les services de santé et les services sociax, Québec: Les Publications du Québec.

Litvak, E. (1985). *Helping the Elderly: The Complementary Roles of Informal Networks and Formal Systems.* New York: Guilford.

McConnell, S. and J. Riggs. (1994). "A Public Policy Agenda: Supporting Family Caregiving" in M. Cantor (ed.), *Family Caregiving: An Agenda for the Future.* San Francisco: American Society on Aging.

Ministère de la santé et des services sociaux. (1988). *Rapport de la Commission d'enquête sur les services de santé et les services sociax,* Québec: Les Publications du Québec.

Ministry of Health and Ministry Responsible for Seniors. (1993). *New Directions for a Healthy British Columbia.* Province of British Columbia.

Moore, S.T. (1991). "Integrating Community Services and Family Care." *Community Alternatives*, 3(1), 33-40.

Neysmith, S. (1991). "From Community Care to a Social Model of Care" in C. Baines, P. Evans and S. Neysmith (eds.), *Women's Caring: Feminist Perspectives on Social Welfare*. Toronto: McClelland and Stewart.

Ontario Office for Seniors Citizens' Affairs. (1986). *A New Agenda: Health and Social Service Strategies for Ontario's Seniors.* Toronto.

Osterbusch, S., S. Keigher, B. Miller and N. Linsk. (1987). Community Care Policies and Gender Justice. *International Journal of Health Services*, 17, 217-232.

Pitrou, A. (1992). *Les solidarités familiales: Vivre sans famille.* Toulouse, France, Editions Privat.

Qureshi, H. and A. Walker. (1989). *The Caring Relationship: Elderly People and Their Families.* Philadelphia, PA: Temple University Press.

Shanas, E. (1979). "The Family: A Social Support System in Old Age." *The Gerontologist,* 19, 3-9.

Statistics Canada. (1996). *Who Cares? Caregiving in the 1990s .* General Social Survey, Ottawa.

Stone, R., G.L. Cafferata and J. Sangl. (1987). "Caregivers of the Frail Elderly: A National Profile." *The Gerontologist*, 27(5), 616-626.

Strawbridge, W.J. and M.I. Wallhagen. (1991). "Impact of Family Conflict on Adult Child Caregivers." *The Gerontologist*, 31, 770-777.

Thurer, S.L. (1983). "Deinstitutionalization and Women: Where the Buck Stops." *Hospital and Community Psychiatry*, 34, 1162-1163.

Waerness, K. (1987). "On the Rationality of Caring," p. 207-234 in A.S. Sassoon (ed.), *Women and the State.* London: Unwin Hyman Inc.

Walker, A. (1987). "Enlarging the Caring Capacity of the Community: Informal Support Networks and the Welfare State." *International Journal of Health Services*, 17(3), 369-386.

——— (1991). "The Relationship Between Family and the State in the Care of Older People." *Canadian Journal of Aging*, 10(2), 94-112.

Webb, A. and G. Wistow. (1987). *Social Work, Social Care and Social Planning: The Personal Social Services Since Seebohm.* London: Longman.

Zarit, S.H. (1991). "Interventions With Frail Elders and Their Families: Are They Effective and Why?" in M.A.P. Stephens, J.H. Crowther, S.E. Hobfoll and D.L. Tannenbaum (eds.), *Stress and Coping in Later-life Families.* New York: Hemisphere.

Zarit, S.H., M.A. Parris Stephens, A. Townsend and R. Greene. (1998). "Stress Reduction for Family Caregivers: Effects of Adult Day Care Use. Journal of Gerontology: Social Sciences, 53B (5), S267-277.

What Research Reveals About Gender, Home Care and Caregiving: Overview and the Case For Gender Analysis

Marika Morris

INTRODUCTION

More than two-thirds of home care[1] recipients are women and the vast majority of unpaid caregivers are women. Beyond the difference in numbers, the experiences of women and men recipients and caregivers vary as a result of male-female differences in socioeconomic status, social roles, lifestyles, physiological and psychological factors and responsibilities. This chapter is based on a review of 45 gender-sensitive research studies on home care and caregiving primarily in Canada,[2] and outlines the differential impact of unpaid caregiving on women and men, in areas such as health, income, employment and benefits, violence in the home, relationships between the recipient and caregiver or other family members, occupational health and safety, stress, isolation and other mental health issues, and expectations of the level of care provided or received. The evidence in this chapter provides a solid structure of knowledge on which to build a gender-based analysis of home care policy and practices.

RESEARCH FINDINGS

Women are the majority of unpaid caregivers and care recipients. According-ing to the Statistics Canada 1996 General Social Survey (GSS) 61 percent of caregivers to seniors with functional limitations were women (Keating et al. 1999). Unfortunately, the data do not include care for persons under 65 with short- or long-term functional limitations.

Seniors with functional limitations are the largest user group of formal and informal home care. According to the 1996 GSS, three-quarters of a million non-institutionalized seniors received assistance because of long-term health problems, whereas data from the National Population Health Survey (NPHS) from 1995 show that 186,500 lived in health care-related institutions. According to a Statistics Canada survey, two-thirds (67 percent) of the community-dwelling seniors receiving paid or unpaid care were women, and 73 percent of residents of health-care-related institutions were women. Paid and unpaid home care allows many people to continue to live in their own homes (Keating et al. 1999).

One reason why women receive more home care could be because they have a longer life expectancy than men and therefore compose the majority of Canada's seniors. Another possible reason is that women play a caregiving role within the family, so when the caregiver herself develops physical or mental limitations, the family seeks outside help. A third reason is that, since women tend to outlive their male partners, they are less likely than men to have a spouse to care for them in old age (Morris, Robinson and Simpson 1999). Lower-income people are also more likely to receive public home care services (Wilkins and Park 1998). The majority of low-income people in Canada are women (Statistics Canada 2000) thus making them more likely than men to be unable to afford private home care services (Morris et al. 1999).

For community-dwelling seniors who received care, 90 percent of assistance with household tasks and errands was provided by unpaid caregivers. Only 10 percent of help with these tasks was provided formally by government or non-government organizations or by a caregiver paid by the senior. Two-thirds of the personal, intimate care tasks were provided by family and friends (Keating et al. 1999).

Women give more hours of care and receive fewer hours of care than men.
Although there are greater numbers of women receiving assistance, they do not receive more hours of care. Female seniors with functional limitations received an average 3.9 hours per week of care, whereas men received 4.9 hours of care. Higher proportions of women seniors than men received no assistance (30 percent compared with 23 percent) which suggests that women are at greater risk of having their needs unmet (Keating et al. 1999).

Women also receive less short-term, post-operative home care than men.
King and Koop (1999) found that the patterns of informal caregiving noted in the chronic care literature are also present in the short-term care of post-surgical cardiac patients. The burden of caregiving continues to rest predominantly on women. Female patients relied on their spouses for help less frequently than did male patients. Thirty percent of caregivers were reported to have a health problem of their own to manage while caring for the recovering patient. Patients who were male or under 65 years of age (either sex) received more support than did patients who were female or 65 years of age or older (either sex). The authors concluded that the cardiac patient's sex affects the availability of home-based care (King and Koop 1999).

Caregivers' employment status affects caregiving. The imbalance between the numbers of female and male caregivers cannot be explained away by who has paid employment. Even when women have paid jobs, many also have unpaid home care responsibilities. One study revealed that 15 percent of women with paid employment and 10 percent of their male counterparts were caregivers (Cranswick 1997). Female caregivers in full-time paid employment performed an average of 4.2 hours of care, whereas their male counterparts gave 2.6 hours. Three-quarters of male caregivers (70.5 percent) and almost half of female caregivers (46.8 percent) had full-time paid employment (Keating et al. 1999).

Fifteen percent of women caregivers were employed part-time, compared with 7.4 percent of male caregivers. The female caregivers who were also employed part-time performed 4.6 hours per week of care on average, while their male counterparts performed an average of 2.3 hours of care (Keating et al. 1999).

Amongst unemployed women and men – that is, those who are actively searching for work, 16 percent of women and 12 percent of men combined their job search activities with caregiving responsibilities (Cranswick 1997).

About 15 percent of women homemakers were caregivers to people with functional limitations. Almost one-fifth of Canadian women can be said to personify the "sandwich generation" – women with both children and elderly or disabled persons to care for. Sixteen percent of women living with a spouse and children were also caregivers of people with functional limitations (Cranswick 1997).

Do men and women who stay at home do an equal share of caregiving? No. Thirty-eight percent of caregiving women were not in the labour force, compared with 22.2 percent of caregiving men. These women provided an average of 6.2 hours per week of care, compared with 5.0 hours for men. Being in paid employment reduced the number of hours of care for both women and men, but more so for men (Keating et al. 1999).

Women with less formal education provide more hours of care. The levels of education of caregivers versus non-caregivers were not significantly different. However, women with lower levels of education tended to provide more hours of care, leading the authors of one national survey to postulate that women with higher levels of education may be in a position to reduce their caregiving hours by purchasing care (Keating et al. 1999). This also has implications for the income, pensions and access to benefits for women who are already lower-income if they give up hours of paid work in order to take on unpaid responsibilities.

Caregiving interferes with ordinary life more for women than men. Women were more likely than male caregivers to feel pressed for time. A higher proportion of female than male caregivers reported having to: make changes in social activities (47 percent versus 44 percent); change holiday plans (26 percent versus 25 percent); postpone plans to enrol in an education or training program (7 percent versus 5 percent); move in with the care recipient (7 percent versus 5 percent); move closer to the person being helped (15 percent versus 9 percent); change sleep patterns (31 percent versus 26 percent) because of the care (Cranswick 1997). The more hours of care women provided, the greater the impact on their lives.

Women travel further and more often than men to provide unpaid care. Joseph and Hallman (1998) revealed a significant relationship between distance from the elder and the average weekly number of hours devoted to eldercare. However, when the data were disaggregated by gender, the study revealed that only male caregivers were less willing to travel in order to care for a distant relative. Women caregivers were willing to travel further and more often than male caregivers, even when the women had paid employment.

More women than men provide more demanding forms of caregiving. According to Kaden and McDaniel (1990) wives and daughters provided the bulk of the more demanding daily and weekly caregiving tasks, whereas husbands and sons were more likely to assist with intermittent, sporadic tasks. Of those who received daily/weekly assistance from spouses, approximately 77 percent was from wives and approximately 24 percent from husbands. Of those who received daily/weekly assistance from offspring, 87 percent was from daughters and 13 percent from sons.

The Canadian Study of Health and Aging (1994) found that seniors who were living in the community and were suffering from dementia were more likely than those without dementia to have a female caregiver (75 percent versus 66 percent). The study found that only 44 percent of the caregivers in the dementia group were satisfied with services provided, versus 95 percent of the caregivers of the group without dementia, and that depressive symptoms were twice as common among the caregivers to persons with dementia.

More women than men are caregivers of multiple persons with functional limitations. We may tend to think of the caregiving relationship as being between only two people – one caregiver and one recipient of care. However, many caregivers perform caregiving responsibilities for multiple persons, and women more so than men. Two-thirds of both the male and female caregivers cared for more than one senior with limitations. Almost 9 percent of female unpaid caregivers of seniors with functional limitations were caring for five or more persons at one time, compared with 5.5 percent of male caregivers (Keating et al. 1999).

Caregiving primarily negatively affects the health of women rather than men. Keating et al. (1999) found that caregiving affected the health of 27.5 percent of female caregivers compared with 10.6 percent of male caregivers. The Roeher Institute (2000) compared the health of mothers of children with disabilities in its sample to the health of mothers in general as measured by the 1996 NPHS. Mothers providing care to children with disabilities were in considerably poorer health. For example, 40 percent of Canadian mothers reported their health as "very good" compared with 12 percent of mothers of children with disabilities. Over half of the mothers in the Roeher sample reported symptoms of stress, including anxiety, depression, disrupted sleep, headaches, isolation, frustration, fear, anger, agoraphobia, hopelessness, feeling overwhelmed, ulcers, fatigue, stomach aches, hypertension and chronic pain. Three-quarters of the mothers said their caregiving role to the child with disabilities caused stress and tension in the family and had an impact on the other siblings. They also reported strains in their marriage and an inability to do things most families take for granted, such as planning holidays. Many of the participants said it was not the child with disabilities who caused stress, it was the lack of adequate community care and support.

In a Manitoba study, daughters were more likely to have higher levels of caregiver burden than sons and employed adult children reported higher levels of burden than those not employed, suggesting that trying to balance employment and caregiving adds to the burden that caregivers experience (Hawranik and Strain 2000).

A British study found that wives as caregivers of spouses with dementia had levels of strain and morale significantly worse than husbands in a similar situation. There were differences between husbands and wives in terms of caregiving tasks. Wives were less able to tolerate the degree to which dementia sufferers depended on them. They were also more likely to wish to leave caregiving to someone else and cited more reasons for wanting to quit. Subjects of both sexes displayed a strong tendency to view women as generally better suited to the caregiving role, and wives felt a greater obligation to care. The authors concluded that attitudinal/social factors were the chief determinants of wives' higher levels of strain and distress, in that they were expected to do more and felt they had less choice in the matter (Collins and Jones 1997).

Turner and Catania (1997) found higher caregiver burden on a specific group of men. They examined persons caring for people with AIDS (PWAs) in a number of U.S. cities. The largest group of caregivers were male friends of the PWA, a group not typically found among caregivers to persons with other types of illnesses. In general, gay or bisexual caregivers, caregivers who had traditional family ties to the PWA, men and lower-income caregivers reported the greatest burden.

Stress was a major factor for caregivers in a large number of gender-sensitive studies. Major stress-related results of caregiving included: family/relationship breakdown (Campbell et al. 1998; Jewitt 1995); abuse (Jewitt 1995); financial insecurity (Campbell et al. 1998; Jewitt 1995; Tremblay et al. 1998); burnout (Campbell et al. 1998; Morris et al. 1999), isolation (Blakley and Jaffe 1999; Campbell et al. 1998; Hawranik and Strain 2000; Roeher Institute 2000); role overload (Jewitt 1995; Keating et al. 1999); and losing one's identity (Campbell et al. 1998).

Other factors included physical/emotional breakdown or illness (Campbell et al. 1998), and the development of specific ailments such as ulcers, headaches, stomach aches, hypertension and chronic pain (Roeher Institute 2000); depression (Blakley and Jaffe 1999; Hibbard et al. 1996; Jewitt 1995; Roeher Institute 2000); exhaustion/fatigue (Blakley and Jaffe 1999; Campbell et al. 1998;

Roeher Institute 2000; Tremblay et al. 1998); sleep disruption (Keating et al. 1999; Roeher Institute 2000; Tremblay et al. 1998); generally deteriorating health (Blakley and Jaffe 1999); and not enough time to engage in caring for their own health and well-being (Blakley and Jaffe 1999; Campbell et al. 1998).

Emotional consequences of stress resulted in feeling overwhelmed (Collins and Jones 1997; Roeher Institute 2000); fear (Campbell et al. 1998); anxiety (Rudd et al. 1999); anger (Jewitt 1995; Keating et al. 1999; Roeher Institute 2000; Rudd et al. 1999); guilt[3] (Blakley and Jaffe 1999; Campbell et al. 1998; Rudd et al. 1999); grief (Jewitt 1995); denial (Jewitt 1995); frustration[4] (Blakley and Jaffe 1999; Campbell et al. 1998; Hawranik and Strain 2000; Roeher Institute 2000); helplessness (Campbell et al. 1998); powerlessness (Blakley and Jaffe 1999); desperation (Campbell et al. 1998); confusion (Campbell et al. 1998), and loneliness (Campbell et al. 1998).

The stress on caregivers is partly due to the finding that home care assessments do not take into account the capabilities and limitations of the caregiver and the family situation. Caregivers are expected to do more than they are able (Campbell et al. 1998; Chapman 1995).

Tremblay et al. (1998) discussed the trend in Quebec towards deinstitution-alization and assigning an increasing number of responsibilities to families, drawing on conceptions of unconditional love, sacrifice and duty. The authors explained that the division of responsibilities along gender lines means women are largely expected to provide personal care for dependents, and are seen as better suited to interpersonal relationships and support. Women thrust into caregiving must develop strategies to handle the multiple pressures of personal life, domestic and family responsibilities, social and professional lives, within a context of inflexible public and private services.

Women have greater support networks, but they are not always helpful. Social support is one of the determinants of health. Hibbard et al. (1996) studied gender differences in the support networks of caregivers. Women tended to have larger social networks, but were also more likely to experience conflict in these networks. Intrafamily conflict is a predictor of caregiver depression. The authors postulated that the sources of conflict were excessive or multiple role demands and the greater provision of personal care by women. The study found that men and women were at risk of insufficient support in different ways: men as a result of insufficient social resources to draw upon, particularly older, lower-income men, and women because of the existence of many sources of conflict.

Some factors contribute to caregivers' well-being. The literature does outline some positive consequences of caregiving. Many caregivers find the work rewarding. Ninety percent of women caregivers to seniors and 86 percent of male caregivers to seniors reported stronger relationships with the care recipient as a result of the caregiving (Keating et al. 1999).

Lauzon et al. (1998) found that the majority of studies dealt with health effects of caregiving, using a theoretical outlook that focused on stress and coping, rather than examining the larger context of the caregiving experience.

The authors highlighted the findings of a few studies with positive findings: that good relationships between the caregiver and the care recipient benefited the caregiver's health, as did supportive relationships in general, recognition from the caregiver's family, the rapid adjustment of the caregiver towards the ethic of caring, attainable goals in caregiving that were respected by health professionals, and ascribing meaning and significance to the caregiving experience. Three strategies identified as being good for caregivers' well-being were: to establish clear limits to caregiving, find a method of reconciling various responsibilities and maximize the potential of the care recipient.

Caregiving interferes with paid work for women more than men. A Statistics Canada survey of caregivers to seniors found that more than half of female caregivers reported that the care had repercussions for their paid work, while less than half of male caregivers reported the same (55 percent versus 45 percent) (Cranswick 1997).

The Roeher Institute (2000) found clear evidence that the caregiving role limits paid labour force participation, economic security and choices of mothers of children with disabilities. Half of the mothers in the survey worked outside the home and 30 percent had full-time paid employment. Those without full-time paid work felt that not working for pay, or working reduced hours, placed an economic strain on the family, but they felt they had little choice. Ninety percent cited their caregiving responsibilities as the reason they could not look for paid work either full-time or part-time. The women working for pay on a part-time basis cited their caregiving responsibilities as their reason for this "choice." One mother was told by her workplace to make a "choice" between her family and her job. Over 50 percent of the mothers had to leave the paid labour force at some point to care for their child with a disability. Over 35 percent had changed jobs or reduced their hours to meet their child's needs. Over 30 percent of the women had encountered difficulties with employers, educators or trainers because they had a child with a disability. Some women looked at their caregiving as a 24-hour-per-day job, and stated that they would have liked some remuneration or recognition. One mentioned worry over her lack of pension after years of caregiving.

Gignac et al. (1996) found that eldercare involvement was significantly associated with interference with paid work for women but not men because women performed eldercare of a different nature and quantity. The women in the sample spent an average of 39.2 hours per week at their paid job and 5.7 hours helping at least one older relative. The men spent an average of 48.3 hours per week at their paid job and 4.9 hours per week assisting an older relative. Women provided more assistance with the activities of daily living. Men's eldercare involvement (for example, help with finances) could more often be dealt with outside of paid work hours. Women reported that family responsibilities resulted in job dissatisfaction and absenteeism.

In a sample of rural caregivers, many had given up paid employment to provide care – fewer than one-quarter held paid employment. Almost half of those who were not currently employed said they had left a paying job or changed jobs because of caregiving responsibilities. The authors calculated that if the caregivers were paid $10.90/hour for the average number of hours they worked, each would receive $92,000 annually (Campbell et al. 1998).

Caregiving involves financial costs for men and women, but more longer-term costs for women. Morris et al. (1999) reported that the financial costs associated with dealing with illness, frailty or disability at home – for example, medical equipment, special meals, renovations to accommodate disabilities, repairs and maintenance in the care setting, and sometimes prescription and non-prescription medications – were largely picked up by recipients, their families and unpaid caregivers and sometimes by paid home care workers. The amount of public funding for these costs vary by jurisdiction.

Cranswick (1997) found that a slightly higher proportion of male than female caregivers reported incurring extra expenses because of the care (46 percent versus 42 percent). However, this tracks the immediate costs related directly to caregiving, rather than the opportunity costs of lost hours of wages, benefits, pension credits, etc.

There are a number of U.S. studies about the cost of informal caregiving, but they do not report the costs by sex. For example, Robinson (1997) found that the estimated annual value of uncompensated care of elderly, ill or disabled relatives in 1990 was US$18 billion and that 9 percent of family caregivers leave the labour force to provide care, 29.4 percent adjust their paid work schedules and 18.1 percent take time off without pay. Thirty-two percent of all family caregivers were poor or near-poor using the U.S. federal poverty level as a measure (Robinson 1997). Arno et al. (1999) measured the market value of the care provided by unpaid family members and friends to ill and disabled adults, estimated at US$196 billion in 1997. This figure substantially exceeds U.S. national spending for formal home health care (US$32 billion) and nursing home care (US$83 billion).

According to Statistics Canada, women perform between CDN$234 billion- CDN$374 billion worth of unpaid work (including housework, child care and elder care) per year in Canada alone (Statistics Canada 1995).

Fast et al. (1997) laid the conceptual groundwork for a Canadian study that would calculate the costs of unpaid caregiving of people with short- or long-term functional limitations, to include costs associated with lost hours of paid employment, pension benefits, missed educational opportunities and other costs in addition to the immediate financial costs of supporting or helping a care recipient. However, Fast et al. (1997) do not consider gender and concentrate only on eldercare.

Armstrong and Kits (2001) outlined the history of state financial support for caregivers. They stated that Nova Scotia provided compensation to caregivers between 1984 and 1994, mainly to young women in rural areas whose "wage" was considerably less than minimum wage for the amount of work they performed. The program was also means-tested. Quebec provides up to $600 to means-tested caregivers to buy respite care. Since 1998, the federal government has offered the Caregiver Tax Credit, which allows a caregiver to claim up to $400 if the claimant's annual income is under $13,853. The authors stated that these programs are inadequate for the needs of caregivers, and benefits delivered through the tax system have little meaning to women whose income is so low there is no taxable income to apply the credit to. The authors also revealed that although some jurisdictions have employment or labour standards legislation that allow short-term and unpaid leave, none require employers to provide caregiver leave. Like a number of other studies, this one pointed out that women's caregiving work in the home is invisible and therefore of less concern to policy-makers.

Mothers are overwhelmingly the primary caregivers of children with disabilities and face special challenges. The Roeher Institute's study of caregivers to children with disabilities – 96 percent of whom were mothers – found that caregivers spent an average of 50-60 hours per week on providing personal care, advocacy, coordination of services and transportation directly related to the child's disability, of which about 3-4 hours per day involved hands-on personal care, such as bathing, feeding, providing medical assistance, etc. Some of the children had high needs and required about 18 hours per day of personal care, some of which was provided by paid workers. One mother spent 17 hours per week just coordinating and advocating support services for her daughter, without counting transportation time to and from programs and appointments. The available services were disjointed and required coordination: The majority of mothers reported involvement in 3-5 community agencies or organizations that supported their children (Roeher Institute 2000).

The Roeher Institute (2000) reported that over 70 percent of the mothers were dissatisfied with the amount of community support they received. Less than 25 percent of the women had any extended family supporting them and, if they did, it tended to be sporadic. Twelve percent of the women felt that if, for whatever reason, they were unable to perform their caregiving role, there would be no one at all to turn to.

Health care cutbacks were also a concern, which the mothers pointed to as the reason why specialized medical and therapeutic services were becoming even more difficult to access. Many health professionals also did not grasp the strain the parents were under, focused on tests and diagnoses rather than the total well-being of the child, and were insensitive – for example, blaming mothers for the disability ("What did you do? Fall? Drink? Paint?") or telling a medical student present in the office, "This child will probably be dead in a year" without having ever previously mentioned the possibility of fatality to the parents (Roeher Institute 2000).

Fullmer et al. (1997) found that most caregivers to adults with mental disabilities were older women and that there was a difference in how they treated daughters and sons with disabilities. Mothers of mentally disabled daughters were more likely to feel burdened by caregiving, even though they received the most help from disabled daughters with household tasks, and were less likely to use day services for their daughters.

Women and men care recipients are subject to violence and physical safety risks, but women caregivers may be at greater risk than men. Elder abuse or abuse of older adults is the "mistreatment of older people by those in a position of trust, power or responsibility for their care," which can include physical, psychological and financial abuse and neglect, which is the failure of a caregiver to meet the needs of an older adult who is unable to meet those needs alone. This includes denial of food, water, medication, medical treatment, therapy, nursing services, health aids, clothing and visitors (Swanson 1998). According to Health Canada, approximately 4 percent of older Canadian adults living in private homes reported experiencing abuse or neglect, but these data are not disaggregated by sex. Information was also not collected or reported about what proportion of these people experienced functional limitations, were receiving paid or unpaid care, and whether they were abused or neglected by paid or unpaid caregivers, or other family members or professionals. The publication reported that males are more likely to be perpetrators of physical abuse and women are more likely to be perpetrators of neglect and financial abuse (Swanson 1998).

Saxton et al. (2001) investigated the perceptions and experiences of women with physical and cognitive disabilities related to abuse by formal and informal personal assistance providers. They found that women with disabilities experienced expanded forms of abuse, and that there was social and personal boundary confusion and power dynamics within the personal assistance services relationship, including with family and friends. The women also experienced personal, social and systemic barriers that impeded their response to abuse. The title of the study ("Bring my scooter so I can leave you") exemplified the dependence many women with disabilities have on care providers, and how difficult it can be to get away from an abusive person on whom one depends for mobility and other forms of assistance with everyday tasks.

Morris et al. (1999) reported that some care recipients had experienced financial abuse and harassment by paid and unpaid caregivers, but had little recourse. A number of studies mentioned that women caregivers are at risk of violence, particularly by care recipients who are mentally ill or with whom there had been a pre-existing family relationship of abuse (Côté et al. 1998; Morris et al. 1999). Although male caregivers may also be at risk of some violence, average physical differences in strength between women and men, and different gender roles about responding to physical violence, may result in more men than women being able to successfully defend themselves against physical attack by a family member being cared for.

Morris et al. (1999) found that care recipients, home care workers and unpaid caregivers all had health, safety and human rights concerns. The physical safety of recipients, paid and unpaid caregivers was at risk due to the overwork and inadequate training of paid and unpaid care providers. Again, because of the average physical strength differences between women and men, the likelihood of injuring oneself while trying to transfer a heavy care recipient from bed to chair may be more significant for women. Unpaid caregivers were not covered under any Workers' Compensation plan if injured at their unpaid job.

Caregivers and recipients in immigrant, refugee and/or visible minority communities face racism, language and cultural barriers. Morris et al. (1999) found that both caregivers and care recipients belonging to visible and linguistic minority groups experienced racism in their access to home care services. For example, one disabled woman of colour was told by her home support worker that, "as an immigrant you should be grateful that you are here and for the services you receive." The authors, who also interviewed home care agency managers, found that there is no mechanism to deal with complaints of racism. There is no anti-racism training provided to home care staff and if any linguistic/racial/ethnic matching of staff to recipients occurs, it does so on an ad hoc basis.

Talbot et al. (1998) conducted interviews with women immigrant family caregivers of Haitian, Asian and Italian origin in Quebec. They found that isolation was compounded by language and cultural differences with main-stream society, and difficulties in negotiating the health care system.

Majumdar et al. (1995) found that non-whites and non-Anglophones were significantly under-represented as clients in three home care agencies in southern Ontario. This points to the possibility that women in these communities may face a greater burden of unpaid care to compensate for fewer paid services and support. Mayatela et al. (1999) found that women perform the role of informal caregiver in 70 to 80 percent of immigrant families. Armstrong and Kits (2001) made an important point about not assuming that ethnic and racial differences in living arrangements for older and disabled relatives are necessarily due to cultural differences rather than low incomes, lack of pensions, lack of access to linguistic and culturally appropriate services, and immigration sponsorship rules.

Aboriginal women caregivers and care recipients are disadvantaged and poorly served. Morris et al. (1999) found that, in recent years, Health Canada has begun to transfer responsibility for health services to some individual Bands. The study found, through interviews with representatives of organizations such as the Aboriginal Nurses of Canada, that home care was not taken into account in the planning of these transfers. Unless Bands had the foresight to specifically ask for home care funds, they were told that no more funds were available. The study also found that, although Aboriginal men and women are affected by early discharge from hospitals like everyone else, home care services are not available on most reserves and remote communities, despite the existence of a limited federal government program. This has two implications for women. The study found that untrained, unpaid women are the home care system in many of these communities and they are expected to provide care in often poor, overcrowded and unhealthy housing conditions, and women, as the majority of care recipients, experience the results of lack of service through transfer to large urban centres, often very far from family and friends, where they are isolated. Métis people and men and women of Aboriginal ancestry who are not "status Indians" are covered by the same provincial programs as other Canadians, but these programs are not culturally sensitive to Aboriginal peoples.

Lesbian and gay caregivers face additional stress and roadblocks. Aronson (1998) interviewed lesbian caregivers of lesbians who needed care by virtue of an illness or disability. She concluded that lesbians live much of their lives outside heterosexual kinship structures and may be less likely to turn to their families for support because of heterosexism or rejection.

Lesbian caregiving can go beyond partners and friends to community networks. The author gave as an example a spontaneous network of support that developed around a Hamilton lesbian with breast cancer. She pointed out that the type of disease or disability might be a factor in the amount of mobilization of support around an individual – for example, breast cancer is highly politicized, whereas someone suffering from chronic fatigue may not be able to build up such a network.

Other factors affecting lesbians included mixed experiences with institutions. Sometimes lesbians were supported and respected, other times not. This led to doubt and anxiety around seeking formal care. Study participants frequently referred to heterosexist bias in the health care system, workplace and legal system as barriers to caregiving. For example, some felt that they could not disclose their true relationship to the person in need of care to health professionals, leading one individual to pass herself off as a sister instead of a partner in order to ensure access to her partner in hospital, or people at work not understanding why the individual was taking so much time off to care for a "friend," or one individual losing a court battle to care for her partner who was physically and cognitively impaired after a car crash because the partner's father objected to the relationship. That lesbians are often poorly treated by institutions places a greater obligation on lesbian partners and friends to care for an individual at home, in order not to expose her to bias and rejection.

Gendered expectations that women will provide unpaid caregiving labour in the family applied to lesbians too. Lesbians' relationships with partners were not taken as seriously as their siblings' commitments to opposite-sex marriages, and so lesbians may be more responsible than heterosexual siblings for caring for their own parents.

Turner and Catania (1997) found that being a gay or bisexual caregiver of a person living with AIDS was a predictor of caregiver burden. It is possible that caring for someone with a stigmatized disease associated with one's own community may be an additional stress factor in caregiving. In a study of U.S. racial minority women living with AIDS, all the caregivers, including men and women, reported the emotional burden of not revealing the HIV/AIDS diagnoses (Baker et al. 1998).

The burden of caregiving is greater for rural women than for urban women or rural men. Female caregivers to seniors with functional limitations provided an average of 4.7 hours of care per week in urban areas and 6.0 hours in rural areas. By contrast, their male counterparts in urban areas provided an average of 3.1 hours per week of care and male rural caregivers provided 2.9 hours (Keating et al. 1999).

Campbell et al. (1998) point out that Canadians living in rural areas tend to have, on average, less education, lower incomes and higher rates of unemployment, illiteracy and dependence on social assistance. Rates of long-term disability and chronic illness are also higher in rural communities than in cities and there is a higher proportion of elderly people in rural Canada. The higher numbers of elderly and disabled Canadians in rural areas coupled with dwindling health services place a greater demand on rural family caregivers. Resources for rural caregivers are minimal to non-existent. Rural areas also tend to be more conservative and traditional, which places an even greater expectation on rural women to fulfill traditional roles as unpaid caregivers. The isolation felt by most caregivers is intensified in rural areas because of a lack of services, transportation and support networks.

According to a Statistics Canada survey, both female and male seniors in failing health who lived in rural areas were statistically more likely to receive assistance than those in cities. The suggested explanation was that seniors in rural areas are more likely to have extensive, closely knit, informal networks and a stronger sense of community (Keating et al. 1999). This is viewed by Blakley and Jaffe (1999) as a stereotype that contributes to the lack of resources for home care in rural areas.

Blakley and Jaffe (1999) discussed the context of the closing of hospitals and long-term care facilities in rural Saskatchewan, the deinstitutionalization of people who are chronically ill or disabled, the scarcity and increasing centralization of respite and physical therapy services, and the shift from hospital to home care. In that province, regional health districts are responsible for home care, and service levels and eligibility vary by district. Some services that would be available at no cost to people receiving care in hospitals is not available free of charge to people receiving care at home. Family caregivers as a stakeholder group are not represented on health district boards and policies that affect them are made without their input. The authors reported that assumptions are made about women being available and suitable for unpaid caregiving work, about strong ties and large families in rural areas when few families today have more than one or two relatives in the community, about financial stability when the financial situation of many rural families is poor, about the lower cost of living in rural areas that does not take into account hidden costs such as transportation, and about rural areas as idyllic settings when they can be isolating and lacking in social resources.

In Blakley and Jaffe's study (1999) almost all the rural women caregivers reported having taken on the role because of a lack of family alternatives: other family members lived too far away or had passed away. Sometimes other family members were unwilling to help because of pre-existing family dynamics, such as the care receiver's alcoholism or the receiver's past abuse or neglect of these family members.

Health care restructuring has particularly hurt women. Armstrong (1996) documented the growing trend of placing the responsibility for health solely on the individual rather than on the medical establishment and society. She pointed out how the language of the women's health movement has been co-opted by government to support withdrawal of intervention: ideas such as self-help, prevention, community settings and reduction of physicians' autonomy, which were designed to give women more control over their health, and reflect a more holistic approach to health have instead been used to justify cutbacks to primary care and the offloading of health care work to mainly women unpaid caregivers.

There has been a great deal of research activity in Quebec about the effects of the shift from hospital to home and community care on women, due to provincial health care reform in the 1990s. Research has come from a variety of sources, including grassroots organizations such as the Coalition féministe pour une transformation du système de santé et des services sociaux (1999); partnerships between grassroots organizations and academics (Côté et al. 1998) and agencies of the Quebec government (Conseil du statut de la femme 2000). They all come to the same conclusion: the shortening of hospital stays, the shift to home and community care, has hurt women as caregivers and care recipients because services are inadequate, under-funded and rely largely on an untrained, unpaid workforce of women who often do not have a choice about whether to provide care.

Aronson and Neysmith (2001) examined the effects on women with disabilities and older women receiving care of the 1996 introduction of "managed competition" in home care in Ontario. Because of minimalist homemaking and personal care services after the reforms, recipients felt apprehensive and ashamed of receiving visitors into their home because of the untidiness of their home and their own unkempt appearance. Most recipients were now entitled to only one bath or shower per week, regardless of how they sweated or smelled, or how poor personal hygiene and appearance made them feel. Reforms meant workers were rushed and unable to provide the social contact that recipients had valued. Changes and discontinuities in providers resulted from shifting contractual arrangements with provider organizations. Recipients experienced a "succession of strangers" entering their homes and privacy, requiring repeated and exhausting explanations of their particular needs and the organization of their homes. Certain tasks that homemakers used to do were now off limits, such as taking out the garbage.

Campbell et al. (1998) also found that some Nova Scotian rural caregivers felt abandoned by the government. It may be that, even if some governments have invested or reinvested in primary health care and/or in community care, these reinvestments have not been sufficient to meet the growing demand. As technology accelerates, life is prolonged both for older people and for children with disabilities, who may not have otherwise lived 50 years ago. In addition to the greater numbers of people who need care, the number of caregivers has diminished due to smaller family sizes and the fact that families are more spread out geographically (Campbell et al. 1998).

Under-funding and insufficient services were also themes in a gender-sensitive study conducted in Manitoba and Newfoundland. Morris et al. (1999) found that care recipients suffered from inadequately funded home care, which led to barriers in access to subsidized care due to tight eligibility requirements, inadequate hours of home care services being assessed (for example, less than the doctor had recommended) and limits on hours of care and types of care. Participants reported that women were sometimes inappropriately assessed for fewer hours of care because of the greater expectation on the part of case managers that older women, women who were ill, and women with disabilities could take better care of themselves than men could. Regional and provincial variations in funding left caregivers and care recipients with unequal access to publicly funded home care. Access to the private purchase of home care depends on income. Older women and women with disabilities tend to have very low incomes and are not able to purchase services. Under-funding of home and community care worked in tandem with insufficient support from other government programs. Inadequate income support programs for older women and women with disabilities, the two largest user groups of publicly funded home care, made these groups extremely vulnerable to poverty which has health and social impacts beyond not being able to cope with the private costs associated with care in the home. Caregivers were not always aware of available respite care services. The female gender role could lead to an underutilization of services even if caregivers were aware of them, as female caregivers might feel guilty about taking time for themselves. Sometimes the fees for these services put them out of the reach of the caregiver, which could be particularly true for female caregivers as there is a statistical gap between women's and men's incomes, leaving women in a poorer economic position to purchase services.

Almost three-quarters of a million community-dwelling seniors received care from family and friends for long-term health problems, compared with 186,500 seniors living in health-care-related institutions (Keating et al. 1999). The provision of unpaid care in the community prevents institutionalization and further costs to government arising from institutionalization, but offloads these costs onto primarily female caregivers and care recipients.

Caregivers, who are predominantly women, and care recipients, who are predominantly older women and women with disabilities, are left out of the policy-making process. A number of studies mentioned that many caregivers believe that governments talk about being "partners" in care, but the caregivers are not listened to (Campbell et al. 1998; Côté et al. 1998; Hawranik and Strain 2000). In a study of frail elderly people receiving care, unpaid family caregivers and paid home care providers, Aronson and Neysmith (1997) pointed out that policy decisions about the design, operation and implementation of long-term care programs have not taken into account the views of those most affected, that is, the frail elderly themselves.

Harlton et al. (1998) interviewed elders, family members, friends and neighbours, volunteers, direct service providers, local and provincial policy-makers and federal policy-makers. They found a marked difference between the views of elders and policy-makers as to who should provide eldercare services. Policy-makers believed that the best care is from unpaid sources close to the older adult. Seniors, on the other hand, said they did not want to "be a burden" on their families and that using public or other paid services allowed them to remain in control.

Aronson and Neysmith (2001) conclude that home care policies are played out in a cultural context in which old age and disability are disparaged, and those who experience it are not viewed as valuable human beings and participants in a democratic society. Care recipients wished to be viewed as citizens, not just service users. The authors made the case for how the dominance of the health care perspective, increasingly market oriented, obscures the fact that these policies are creating or reinforcing the social exclusion of women with disabilities and older women from our society.

ANALYSIS AND CONCLUSION

Why do women form the majority of caregivers? The consensus is that women are socialized and viewed by society as "natural" caregivers and feel pressure to do this work for free (or rather, at their own expense). Women and men experience different socioeconomic contexts and gender-role expectations, which result in women giving more hours of unpaid care than men do, performing more demanding forms of caregiving than men, travelling further and more often to provide unpaid care, and being more likely to have responsibility for more than one care recipient, sacrificing more of their paid work time to perform unpaid care, and feeling obligated by their social role to provide unpaid care. Women and men care recipients are subject to violence and physical safety risks, but women caregivers may be at greater risk than men.

Not surprisingly, research shows that caregiving primarily negatively affects the health of women rather than men, and interferes with women's ordinary lives and plans much more so than men's. The personal and financial costs of caregiving are high, particularly for women. Certain groups of caregivers are particularly poorly served by public systems and face additional burdens: immigrant, refugee and/or visible minority women, Aboriginal women, lesbians and rural women.

Armstrong and Kits (2001) produced an overview of the history of caregiving in the twentieth century. According to the authors, the century was characterized by the entry of married women into the paid labour force; smaller, more mobile families reflecting access to birth control; rising female labour force participation; and divorce. This has had an impact on women's availability to provide unpaid care. Formal health care services expanded, improved and became publicly funded which, along with improved nutrition, housing, income, sanitary and employment conditions, ensured that more people with a disability survived and more people lived into old age. This has meant there are more people for whom to provide care than in the past. New chronic diseases appeared through the century, such as HIV/AIDS and Alzheimer's, as some acute infectious diseases disappeared. This has also led to an increase in demand for long-term care. New technologies and a move to cost-cutting in the later part of the century resulted in deinstitutionalization, and an unprecedented number of people cared for in the home, in unprecedented ways. Throughout these massive changes, the one thing that remained constant was women's responsibility for unpaid caregiving.

A number of studies based in different parts of the country have come to the same conclusion – that health care restructuring has particularly hurt women. Shorter hospital stays, deinstitutionalization and the shift towards community care have added to the burden of unpaid caregiving that women are expected to take on. Health care restructuring has also hurt care recipients, a significant proportion of whom are low-income women who cannot afford to purchase private services when publicly-funded services are inadequate. A pattern emerges of cost-cutting as the primary consideration, over the health, well-being and democratic inclusion of primarily female citizens.

The finding that women care recipients consistently receive fewer hours of care from informal caregivers is a concern (Keating et al. 1999). The needs of women recipients of care may be going unmet, perhaps because it is assumed by care assessment officials and unpaid caregivers that they can take better care of themselves than men. Home care policies and systems must become gender-sensitive to ensure that women with functional limitations are receiving the care they need and that expectations, stereotypes and familiarity with female gender roles are not interfering with women's ability to access care.

The bulk of the home and community care literature does not take gender into account. Sometimes, studies will mention in passing that the majority of caregivers are women or, less often, that the majority of care recipients are women, but will not proceed to do any gender analysis with their data, possibly assuming that caregivers have a uniform experience and that gender does not matter. Or the gender issue will be recognized, but there are no concrete recommendations that deal with it. This is unfortunately the case in the highly publicized Romanow Commission (the Commission on the Future of Health Care in Canada). The Romanow report's 18-page chapter on home care mentions women twice, once to say that the burden on informal caregivers is great, especially for women. The other time was to mention that many presenters to the Commission were concerned about the burden on women (Romanow 2002). The Commission makes no specific mention of women in its home care recommendations, and does not mention women as recipients of care. It suggests the alleviation of informal caregivers' burden through a special leave administered through the Employment Insurance (EI) program. What it fails to mention, as there is no evidence that a gender analysis was performed, is that fewer women than men qualify for EI. A basic gender analysis would reveal that, in 1999, 41 percent of employed Canadian women were "non-standard workers," that is, temporary workers, part-time workers, self-employed persons with no paid staff, and multiple job holders, compared with 29 percent of men (Statistics Canada 2000). As such, women have less access to EI benefits, particularly since recent restrictions on entry. Over a six-year period, the number of women receiving EI benefits has dropped by half (Statistics Canada 2000). A family care leave through EI would benefit some women but exclude many others, particularly workers in more precarious, usually lower-income, types of employment. Also, the Commission does not mention that EI benefits have been slashed to 55 percent of one's salary. Women make up the majority of minimum wage workers in Canada (Statistics Canada 1998). Living on the full minimum wage is an enormous challenge. Living on nearly half of the minimum wage is impossible. Solutions that are proposed without regard to the realities of women's lives and without any gender analysis of their implications are no solutions at all.

Some studies which do go as far as to take gender into account both in data collection and analysis fall short in terms of passing the tests of gender-sensitive research, as they may suffer from a lack of familiarity with previous gender-sensitive work and perspectives that might have informed the research. For example, Hooker et al. (2000) found that wives who cared for husbands with Alzheimer's (AD) reported significantly worse mental health outcomes than husbands, while wives and husbands in the Parkinson's (PD) group showed no differences. They also found that AD caregiving wives were less likely than husbands to use "problem-focused coping strategies." The authors concluded that the loss of reciprocity in marital relationships may affect women more negatively than men (Hooker et al. 2000). If the authors had taken into account previous research that shows a marked difference in the volume and type of duties between caregiving women and men, and that constant care may be necessary for someone living with AD, this might have suggested another variable to look at in this study, which in turn might have had a significant impact on the results and interpretation of the data. Gender-based analysis is not only about counting women and men, or factoring sex/gender as a variable. Women who are putting in more hours, performing more difficult care, at greater risk of violence and exhaustion, are not necessarily in any shape to engage in "problem-focused coping strategies." Gender-based analysis must include becoming familiar with the findings of gender-based research, which can then guide a researcher/analyst towards asking the right questions, and taking the socioeconomic differences and different life experiences of women and men into account when conducting or interpreting research.

Gender-sensitive studies lead us to different and valuable conclusions from research that is not gender-sensitive. For example, by lumping together women and men caregivers in one study, one may conclude that the burden of caregiving is not that great. One may find that caregivers' health is adequate and that caregivers are not severely financially or personally impacted by caregiving. When one separates male from female in studies, a different picture emerges: one group does much less, and caregiving does not have as great an impact on this group, and one group does much more, and the health and long-term financial effects are severe. Research that is not gender-sensitive can therefore underestimate caregiver burden and health, personal and financial impacts, because the one-third of caregivers who are men tend not to give as many hours of care, and give up less in terms of their career and personal life.

Since gender-sensitive research tends to be performed by researchers with a grasp of socioeconomic gender differences, it tends to pay more attention to issues of income and poverty. These studies ask the questions about financial implications, which are reflected in recommendations such as providing a travel allowance/transportation assistance; reviewing income support, disability-related programs, and tax programs to alleviate poverty; establishing workplace policies that take caregiving into account; compensating caregiving work through tax relief, pension benefits, a wage, or some form of financial compensation; timely, appropriate and low-cost respite care; and including counselling services for caregivers and recipients as part of free and available services. This is a perspective that is missing in the mainstream health care debates about user fees, for example. That debate centres around how the government can afford care. What is missing is the gendered perspective of how women afford to continue giving more and more unpaid care and access a health system on low wages or no wages.

Gender-sensitive research brings out how men and women are treated differently as care recipients, something completely lost in research that ignores gender. This has policy implications for the home care assessment process.

Sometimes what is valuable about gender-sensitive research is the perspective of researchers, which tends to consider issues of social justice. These researchers bring up issues such as the citizenship rights of caregivers and recipients. In most of the literature, care recipients in particular tend to be viewed as objects of care, rather than human beings with social and political rights. The majority of care recipients are women seniors and women with disabilities, and another common view is that they are sexless, which leads to an underestimation of how they suffer from violence against women. Gender-sensitive studies stress the importance of involving caregivers and recipients in decision-making at local, provincial and federal levels, which can only lead to more responsive, reality-based policy.

Gender-sensitive research does not just provide answers, it also asks the tricky questions, such as a series of questions developed by Armstrong and Kits (2001) to apply to all policy, legislation and regulations. As women and men experience different socioeconomic contexts, policy decisions about the following have a different impact on women and men who are care recipients and/ or caregivers: which services are publicly funded; assumptions about the type and level of care to be provided by family members or other unpaid caregivers; coverage for out-of-pocket expenses, including drugs, medical supplies, assistive devices, and therapies; and the degree of attention to the needs of caregivers as well as care recipients, including physical and mental health and opportunity costs such as loss of employment.

Hooyman and Gonyea (1995) gave an overview of the history of feminist politicization of unpaid care and attempted to change the discourse about home and community care from an issue of individual maladaptation that tinkering with policy could fix, to one of structural inequality, requiring a transformation of policy and society. The authors pointed out that even studies that recognize caregiving as a women's issue tend to highlight subjective stress and caregiver burden, and result in recommendations involving coping methods, such as education, counselling and social support, and incremental changes in service delivery models. The authors stated that, "the overriding issue is not how to relieve individual stress but how to organize society to achieve gender justice so that care for dependent populations across the life span is more equitable and humane for both those who give and those who receive care.... From a policy perspective, feminists are now questioning how services for adults with disabilities can be offered in ways that do not rely primarily on women to do either the unpaid or underpaid work of caring" (1995:20).

The purpose of gender-based analysis is to develop good, *evidence-based* policy based on a complete picture of how women and men are affected. If home and community care policies are not to entrench and exacerbate gender inequality, they must take into account gender differences and perspectives.

Notes

1. Home care can take multiple forms and be provided by paid professionals and workers, unpaid volunteers sent by organizations such as support agencies for people with particular illnesses or conditions, faith groups or other organizations, or unpaid family members and friends. Keating et al. (1999) state that unpaid caregiving can include medical care, assistance with personal and bodily care, assistance with housework, maintenance, finances, errands and decision-making. They posited that routine assistance becomes "care" when the assistance is compensating for functional loss. For example, concern and lending a hand become "care" when the individual's health problem or disability necessitates that aid be given.

2. The information contained in this chapter is based in part on *Gender-Sensitive Home and Community Care Research: A Synthesis Paper*, December 2001, a report funded by Health Canada. The views expressed herein are not necessarily those of the Government of Canada. A licence was obtained from Health Canada for the use of this material for the purposes of this book chapter.

3. Guilt was a factor for a number of caregivers – guilt over giving birth to a child with disabilities, guilt over being healthy when the other person is ill, guilt about not understanding the other person's illness, guilt over not making the right choices about medications, health professionals or the use of health facilities (Blakley and Jaffe 1999).

4. Factors contributing to frustration were dealing with a "maze of bureaucracy" (Campbell et al. 1998), the denial on the part of function-impaired elders that they needed help (Hawranik and Strain 2000), and the demanding and repetitive nature of caregiving tasks (Blakley and Jaffe 1999).

References

Armstrong, Pat (ed.). (1996). *Unravelling the Safety Net: Transformations in Health Care and Their Impact on Women.* Edited by J. Brodie, *Women and Canadian Public Policy.* Toronto: Harcourt Brace.

Armstrong, Pat and Olga Kits. (2001). "One Hundred Years of Caregiving." Ottawa: Law Commission of Canada.

Arno, P.S., C. Levine and M.M. Memmott. (1999). "The Economic Value of Informal Caregiving." *Health Affairs,* 18 (2):182-188.

Aronson, Jane. (1998). "Doing Research on Lesbians and Caregiving: Disturbing the Ideological Foundations of Family and Community Care" in J. Ristock and C. Taylor (eds.), *Inside the Academy and Out: Lesbian/Gay/Queer Studies and Social Action.* Toronto: University of Toronto Press.

Aronson, Jane and Sheila Neysmith. (1997). "The Retreat of the State and Long-term Care Provision: Implications for Frail Elderly People, Unpaid Family Carers and Paid Home Care Workers." *Studies in Political Economy,* 53 (Summer).

————(2001). "Manufacturing Social Exclusion in the Home Care Market." *Canadian Public Policy/ Analyse de politiques,* 26 (2):151-165.

Baker, S., M. Sudit and E. Litwak. (1998). "Caregiver Burden and Coping Strategies Used by Informal Caregivers of Minority Women Living With HIV/AIDS." *Association of Black Nursing Faculty Journal,* 9 (3):56-60.

Blakley, Bonnie and JoAnn Jaffe. (1999). *Coping as a Rural Caregiver: The Impact of Health Care Reforms on Rural Women Informal Caregivers.* Winnipeg: Prairie Centre of Excellence for Women's Health.

Campbell, Joan, Gail Bruhm and Susan Lilley. (1998). *Caregivers' Support Needs: Insights from the Experiences of Women Providing Care in Rural Nova Scotia.* Halifax: Maritime Centre of Excellence for Women's Health.

Canadian Study of Health and Aging. (1994). "Patterns of Caring for People with Dementia in Canada." *Canadian Journal on Aging/La Revue canadienne du vieillissement,* 13 (4):470-487.

Chapman, Marian. (1995). Panel discussion for community supports (for caregivers of seniors). Paper read at Women as Family Caregivers Symposium. Conference proceedings of the National Council of Women of Canada, l'Association féminine d'éducation et action sociale, Mothers Are Women, and the Canadian Home Economics Association, November 24-26, at Ottawa.

Coalition féministe pour une transformation du système de santé et des services sociaux. (1999). *Attention! Virage dangerux pour la santé des femmes. Rapport des forums interrégionaux sur le virage ambulatoire et la transformation du réseau.* Montréal: L'R des centres de femmes du Québec.

Collins, C. and R. Jones. (1997). "Emotional Distress and Morbidity in Dementia Carers: A Matched Comparison of Husbands and Wives." *International Journal of Geriatric Psychiatry,* 12 (12):1168-1173.

Conseil du statut de la femme. (2000). *Pour un virage ambulatoire qui respecte les femmes.* Québec: Gouvernement du Québec.

Côté, Denyse, Éric Gagnon, Claude Gilbert, Nancy Guberman, Francine Saillant, Nicole Thivierge and Marielle Tremblay. (1998). *Qui donnera les soins? Les effets du virage ambulatoire et des mesuresd d'économie sociale sur les femmes du Québec.* Ottawa: AFÉAS et Condition féminine Canada.

Cranswick, K. (1997). "Canada's Caregivers." *Canadian Social Trends* (Winter).

Fast, Janet E., Norah C. Keating and L. Oakes. (1997). *Conceptualizing and Operationalizing the Costs of Informal Elder Care.* Ottawa: National Health Research Development Program.

Fullmer, E.M., S.S. Tobin and G.C. Smith. (1997). "The Effects of Offspring Gender on Older Mothers Caring for Their Sons and Daughters With Mental Retardation." *Gerontologist,* 37 (6):795-803.

Gignac, Monique, Kevin Kelloway and Benjamin Gottlieb. (1996). "The Impact of Caregiving on Employment: A Mediation Model of Work-Family Conflict." *Canadian Journal on Aging/La Revue canadienne du vieillissement,* 15 (4):525-542.

Harlton, Shauna-Vi, Norah Keating and Janet Fast. (1998). "Defining Eldercare for Policy and Practice: Perspectives Matter." *Family Relations*, 47 (3):1-8.

Hawranik, Pamela and Laurel Strain. (2000). *Health of Informal Caregivers: Effects of Gender, Employment and Use of Home Care Services*. Winnipeg: Prairie Women's Health Centre of Excellence.

Hibbard, J, A. Neufeld and M.J. Harrison. (1996). "Gender Differences in the Support Networks of Caregivers." *Journal of Gerontological Nursing*, 22 (9):15-23.

Hooker, K., M. Manoogian-O'Dell, D.J. Monahan, L.D. Frazier and K. Shifren. (2000). "Does Type of Disease Matter? Gender Differences Among Alzheimer's and Parkinson's Disease Spouse Caregivers." *Gerontologist*, 40:568-573.

Hooyman, Nancy R. and Judith G. Gonyea. (1995). *Feminist Perspectives on Family Care: Policies for Gender Justice*. Thousand Oaks, CA: Sage.

Jewitt, Christine. (1995). Panel discussion on community supports (for caregivers of the adult disabled). Paper read at Women as Family Caregivers Symposium, Conference proceedings of the National Council of Women of Canada, l'Association féminine d'éducation et action sociale, Mothers Are Women and the Canadian Home Economics Association, November 24-26, 1995, at Ottawa.

Joseph, A.E. and B.C. Hallman. (1998). "Over the Hill and Far Away: Distance as a Barrier to the Provision of Assistance to Elderly Relatives." *Social Science & Medicine* 46(6):631-39.

Kaden, Joan and Susan McDaniel. (1990). "Care Giving and Care-receiving: A Double Bind for Women in Canada's Aging Society." *Journal of Women and Aging*, 2 (3):3-26.

Keating, Norah, Janet Fast, Judith Frederick, Kelly Cranswick and Cathryn Perrier. (1999). *Eldercare in Canada: Context, Content and Consequences*. Ottawa: Health Canada.

King, K.M., and P.M. Koop. (1999). "The Influence of the Cardiac Surgery Patient's Sex and Age on Care Giving Received." *Social Science & Medicine*, 48 (12):1735-1742.

Lauzon, Sylvie, Jacinthe Pépin, Maria Elisa Montejo, Jean-Pierre Lavoie and Marlène Simard. (1998). *Bilan critique des études menées sur les expériences des aidantes naturelles à partir d'une perspective émique*. Montréal: Centre d'excellence pour la santé des femmes.

Majumdar, B., G. Browne and J. Roberts. (1995). "The Prevalence of Multicultural Groups Receiving In-home Service from Three Community Agencies in Southern Ontario: Implications for Cultural Sensitivity Training." *Canadian Journal of Public Health*, 86 (3):206-211.

Mayatela, Rose-Marie, Angela Stoica and Lynda Bouthillier. (1999). *Vieillir en contexte migratoire*. Montréal: ACCESSS – Alliance des communautés culturelles pour l'égalité dans la santé et les services sociaux.

Morris, Marika, Jane Robinson and Janet Simpson. (1999). *The Changing Nature of Home Care and its Impact on Women's Vulnerability to Poverty*. Ottawa: Status of Women Canada.

Robinson, K.M. (1997). "Family Caregiving: Who Provides the Care, and at What Cost?" *Nursing Economics*, 15 (5):243-247.

Roeher Institute. (2000). *Beyond the Limits: Mothers Caring for Children with Disabilities*. North York, Ont.: L'Institut Roeher Institute.

Romanow, Roy. (2002). *Building on Values: The Future of Health Care in Canada*. Ottawa: Commission on the Future of Health Care in Canada.

Rudd, M.G., L.L. Viney and C.A. Preston. (1999). "The Grief Experienced by Spousal Caregivers of Dementia Patients: The Role of Place of Care of Patient and Gender of Caregiver." *International Journal of Aging and Human Development*, 48 (3):217-240.

Saxton, Marsha, Mary-Ann Curry, Laurie Powers, Susan Maley, Karyl Eckels and Jacqueline Gross. (2001). "Bring my Scooter so I Can Leave You: A Study of Disabled Women Handling Abuse by Personal Assistance Providers." *Violence Against Women*, 7 (4):393-417.

Statistics Canada. (1995). "Unpaid Work of Households." *The Daily* (Dec 20).

––––––– (1998). *The Daily* (25 August).

––––––– 2000. *Women in Canada 2000: A Gender-based Statistical Report*. Ottawa: Minister of Industry.

Swanson, Susan. (1998). *Abuse and Neglect of Older Adults*. Ottawa: National Clearinghouse on Family Violence, Health Canada.

Talbot, Lise, Olivette Soucy and Luciana Soave. (1998). *Vers l'utilisation des services de réadaption adaptés aux familles multi-éthniques dont une personne présente une défiance motrice ou sensorielle*. Montréal: Centre d'excellence pour la santé des femmes.

Tremblay, Marielle, Nicole Bouchard, Claude Gilbert, Martine Couture, Guylaine Boivin, Hélène Roberge, Marlène Simard and Nicole L'Heureux. (1998). *Les aidantes naturelles et la prise en charge de personnes en perte d'autonomie : santé des femmes et défi des solidarités familiales et sociales*. Montréal: Centre d'excellence pour la santé des femmes.

Turner, H.A. and J.A. Catania. (1997). "Informal Caregiving to Persons With AIDS in the United States: Caregiver Burden Among Central Cities Residents Eighteen to Forty-nine Years Old." *American Journal of Community Psychology*, 25 (1):35-59.

Wilkins, Kathryn and Evelyn Park. (1998). "Home Care in Canada." *Health Reports*, 10 (1).

Redefining Home Care for Women With Disabilities: A Call for Citizenship

Kari Krogh

INTRODUCTION

For disabled women, home care is more than the provision of assistance that facilitates physical or emotional well-being, it is an essential prerequisite for achieving full citizenship. Without formal and informal home care, women with disabilities cannot access the world and engage in their communities. Specifically, many women with long-term impairments require assistance with bathing, dressing and eating before they can attend class, go to work, participate in a community event or go out dancing with a friend.

In this chapter, I will explore ways that gender issues intersect with home care and home care policy to affect the lives of women with long-term impairments. I will focus on home care in the form of general personal assistance, personal hygiene or grooming, housework, meal preparation, errands and informal health monitoring over the long term rather than medical and rehabilitative interventions or other therapies associated with post-acute care discharge from hospital. Many people with disabilities prefer to refer to such home care services as personal assistance or attendant care, emphasizing its location outside of the home, or home support to indicate its non-medical nature. For the purposes of this chapter I will use home care and home support interchangeably.

Home support can enable people with disabilities to move through various physical, social, economic and political spaces to achieve their personal goals. For example, it might include assisting someone who has a mobility impairment in navigating within the home, neighbourhood, campus and pool to achieve goals related to personal health, socialization, education or employment.

I provide a definition of disability according to the central debates within the field of disability studies, supporting a social model analysis that goes beyond physical or mental impairment to the social, political and economic forces that in effect create disabling barriers. I also recognize the value of a phenomenological description of the impairment experience in understanding issues such as fluctuations in levels of impairment and, consequently, care needs. Both these approaches can inform the ways that home support is understood in the lives of people with disabilities and ultimately assist in putting forward policy recommendations that would improve the lives of disabled women. I will draw on data I have collected as a researcher of home care from the perspectives of people with disabilities (e.g., Krogh 2001a, 2001b; Krogh et al. 2003; Krogh and the Home Support Action Group, 2000; Krogh, Johnson and Bowman, 2003). I will also incorporate what I have learned through my engagement with the disability community where the analysis is important but not always gendered. Finally, I will draw indirectly from my own experiences of providing and receiving care as a disabled woman.

Home care is a gendered issue (see, for example, Morris 2001) and disability, like other forms of disadvantage, adds an additional interwoven layer of complexity to the analysis. Women are more likely than men to need care and less likely to receive the level of assistance that they require (Roeher Institute, 1995; Statistics Canada 2001a). Impairments related to mobility are more common in women as are chronic illnesses (Statistics Canada 2001b). Women frequently have their experiences dismissed and their need for assistance denied when they present less visible impairments such as pain and fatigue that are commonly associated with chronic conditions such as rheumatoid arthritis or fibromyalgia (Council of Canadians with Disabilities 2001; Masuda 1998). Society's values are reflected in assessment procedures that not only act as part of a system of surveillance but also frequently render these women ineligible and unworthy of subsidized home care. Many women who live with long-term impairments also live with the effects of gender socialization and are expected to adopt and maintain caregiving roles even when these responsibilities clearly have a negative impact on their health (see, for example, Katz et al. 2000). With the exception of studies on older women and papers written by disabled women, an examination of the role of women with impairments in providing care is notably absent in the published literature.

Women with disabilities who require home care face inequities in society that may be complicated and reinforced by oppression based on, for example, economic status, sexual orientation or race. They are underrepresented in the workforce (Fawcett 1996) and yet they are often not provided with the level of home care assistance that would enable them to receive an education, job training or volunteer experience. Women with and without disabilities form a web of interactions and are affected by the powerful forces of globalization, privatization and regional as well as national health and caregiving policy. It is critical that a feminist analysis of home care acknowledge and include a disability perspective. I propose that disability issues are ultimately women's issues. The category of "disabled" is frequently used to make us distinct, separate and other. As a challenge to this, I invite women to recognize their current or future embodied connection to the terms "disabled," "care provider" and "care recipient."

One woman, whom I interviewed as part of a research study I coordinated on the impact of home care in the lives of people with disabilities, described how the meaning of home care differs for each person receiving care: "We are people who are still trying to live our lives, both before [and] even when we get to be seniors with disabilities ... [we are] university students or professors or activists, we're television watchers, we're people who want to run marathons.... I need people helping me ... it took a lot of fight to get us out of institutions ... to maintain our independence and freedom.... What is independence? What does it look like – it's different for everybody" (Krogh, 2001a).

A SOCIAL MODEL OF DISABILITY

Defining the Social Model of Disability

The way society defines disability has profound implications for how health and home care issues, health policy and policy participation are understood and approached. A social or sociopolitical model of disability has been presented by disability rights activists and academics within the emerging discipline of disability studies. It is presented here in an effort to locate home care for women with disabilities outside of a medical framework.

Barnes, Mercer and Shakespeare (1999:31) in their book, *Exploring Disability: A Sociological Introduction*, described the social model as follows:

> The social model focuses on the experience of disability, but not as something which exists purely at the level of individual psychology, or even interpersonal relations. Instead, it considers a wide range of social and material factors and conditions, such as family circumstances, income and financial support, education, employment, housing, transport and the built environment, and more besides. At the same time, the individual and collective conditions of disabled people are not fixed, and the experience of disability therefore also demonstrates an "emergent" and temporal character. This spans the individual's experience of disability, in the context of their overall biography, social relationships and life history, the wider circumstances of disabling barriers and attitudes in society, and the impact of the state policies and welfare supports systems.

The social model of disability or the sociopolitical formulation of disability was characterized by Rioux (1997:105) as follows:

1. disability is assumed not to be inherent to the individual independent of the social structure;
2. priority is given to the political, social and built environment;
3. secondary rather than primary prevention is emphasized;
4. disability is recognized as difference rather than as an anomaly;

5. disability is viewed as the interaction of individuals with society;
6. inclusion of people with disabilities is seen as a public responsibility;
7. the unit of analysis is the social structure; and
8. the points of intervention are the social, environmental and economic systems.

Transforming the Medical Model of Disability

This framework represents an important challenge to the medical model of disability which has dominated, and continues to dominate, the lives of disabled women and men by constructing them as clients or patients in need of improvement through treatment, surgery, rehabilitation or remediation. The social model locates communities, institutions and governments within society as sites where impairment (i.e., functional difference) is transformed into disability (i.e., oppression or barriers) and thus identifies society as the central place of intervention. Essential concepts within the home care debate are, in effect, transformed through this paradigmatic shift. Terms such as care, control, expertise, professional dominance and personal problem are transformed into rights, choice, experience, individual and collective responsibility, and social problem. Within this model of disability, the focus becomes the social pathology (e.g., structures) with an emphasis on elimination of systemic barriers (e.g., choice in care options) as well as the provision of political and social entitlements (e.g., reformulation of social policy) (see Rioux 1997).

Researchers and government departments such as Human Resources Development Canada (HRDC) are increasingly recognizing the role of environment in the creation of disability. This is reflected to some extent, for example, in the Participation and Activity Limitation Survey (PALS) that defines a person with disability as someone who reports difficulties with daily living activities, or who indicated that a physical or mental condition or health problem reduced the kind or amount of activities in which they could participate (Statistics Canada 2001b). The World Health Organization's (2001) new framework, the International Classification of Functioning, Disability and Health (ICF) examines the body, in addition to individual activities, social participation and social environments, and recognizes the role of environmental factors in either facilitating functioning (body functions, activities and participation) or raising barriers (see the Human Resource Development Canada's [2002] report, "Advancing the Inclusion of People with Disabilities").

A focus on impairment is problematic because it can be seen to emphasize a medical model of disability that focuses on the body while diverting attention away from political targets such as policy. Members of our society automatically assume a correlation between health and the perfect body. The discourse of the perfect body reveals and reinforces how society understands health in relation to disability. The differently abled or impaired body is assumed to be unhealthy when this would not necessarily be the case – there are, in fact, many people with impairments who experience good health in relation to their own standards or norms (Tighe 2001). While people with disabilities expect and desire good health care, they challenge the use of the medical model and notions of the perfect body in a discussion of home care.

This concern can be seen to be consistent with what Hooyman and Gonyea (1999:165-166) present as a feminist model of health. In their opinion, "in a feminist model, health is not just an individual personal problem, but also the responsibility of community and government . . . [and] requires a strong public sector presence that takes leadership in defining policy directions to insure entitlement to health care based on rights of citizenship." This focus on citizenship is central to the disability analysis of home care policy. People who live with long-term impairments not only have insights related to their own bodies, they also have knowledge of ways to navigate through society to achieve their personal goals. Home support, when shaped by people with disabilities themselves, can enable full citizenship. However, this requires flexibility in service delivery, an acceptance of the active role of people with disabilities in society and sufficient resources.

MAKING SPACE FOR IMPAIRMENT AND THE COMPLEXITY OF CHRONIC ILLNESS

Phenomenology and the Social Model of Disability

Within the disability studies arena and the disability movement there has been criticism that an emphasis on the social model has left little space for the phenomenological articulation of the experience of impairment. This is an issue of particular concern for women with disabilities, including those requiring home care, who wish to acknowledge and describe their bodily experience and not deny this as part of being fully human. In fact, women with chronic illness challenge the notion that oppression is experienced solely within social structures (and thus outside the body) when they describe the physicality of having their emotional and physical energy drained by particular interactions relating to evaluation of their home care eligibility.

There is a risk that descriptions of bodily pain may actually contribute to rather than challenge society's notions that equate disability with pain, sickness and tragedy (Clare 1999; Wendell 2001). For women with long-term impairments, there is a concern that overmedicalization of their circumstances will cause the general public and health administrators to believe they need to reside in a long-term care institution when non-medical and community-based personal assistance is what they know they need (Snow 1992). Even worse, a focus on the experience of impairment could be misconstrued to justify acts of murder to end suffering as in the highly publicized instance of Tracy Latimer, the twelve-year-old Canadian girl with cerebral palsy who was killed by her father (Malhotra, 2001). Women with disabilities wish to be free to describe their bodily experiences and the challenges associated with the ongoing reassessment of the body within various social, physical and political spaces. Women with disabilities also wish to be free to publicly celebrate their bodies and their lives as worth living. Disabled feminists such as Jenny Morris (2001) question why the social model cannot be adhered to while also making room for a description of the ways in which impairments affect women's lives. Women who live with impairments are calling for a reconsideration of disability in a manner that acknowledges the struggles within the impaired body enmeshed within a social world.

Women are more likely than men to be impaired by a chronic illness such as multiple sclerosis, rheumatoid arthritis, chronic fatigue immune dysfunction syndrome, depression and fibromyalgia (Trypuc 1994; Wendell 2001). It is important that descriptions of living with these impairments are available to build an understanding of how women's daily tasks are or are not accomplished and supported through home care. The impairments that commonly accompany chronic illness include pain, fatigue and memory difficulties. These forms of impairment last over six months and are less visible than other forms of impairment. Such conditions can also go into remission and then recur or fluctuate from day-to-day or change considerably over time, particularly if the condition is degenerative (Wendell 1996; 2001). Those who have multiple impairments including seasonal affective disorder may find that their need for personal supports follows a seasonal cycle. These types of impairments do not fit easily into home care assessment instruments and procedures – they are difficult to measure objectively and are impossible to separate from women's everyday bodily experience. Evaluators responsible for assessing eligibility for home care are often charged with the task of compartmentalizing symptoms within the body and rating impairment levels as if they are static.

Marginalization of Chronic Illness

Those who implement the assessment of need may lack knowledge of such conditions and question, "Why should you receive assistance? You certainly don't look disabled" (Rhonda Wiebe, a recipient of home care services, personal communication, 4 April, 2003). Applying a Foucauldian analysis, the "gaze" of the home care assessor or administrator legitimizes the application of power over women with disabilities while excluding alternative interpretations (Foucault 1973; 1977). Women who face this form of discrimination would benefit from advocacy support from consumer-directed organizations. This is not always easy, given that chronic illness has been marginalized within the disability community. For example, Humphrey (2000) found that the propensity to consider only tangible impairments as evidence of a genuine disability clearly marginalizes those with nonapparent impairments while bolstering the claim of those with a visible impairment that they represent all disabled people. Further, women with these forms of impairment are frequently considered lazy, slackers, malingerers, uncooperative, hypochondriacs, or otherwise inadequate (Wendell 2001; Young 2000). Constructing women disabled by chronic illness in these ways functions to delegitimate their requests for assistance.

The value-laden gaze has increasingly been used to "scale bodies" against biological norms to determine social acceptability. Disability is ultimately a matter of degree – the bureaucratic and arbitrary line that is drawn between disabled and not disabled enough in order to determine eligibility for service is based on what Young (2000:170-171) and others have called a "politics of resentment" that motivates certain people, including health system administrators, to draw that line as far down the extreme end of the continuum as possible. This operates to build an expectation that people with disabilities will legally conform to certain socially constructed norms.

Embodiment and Home Care Assessment

Helen Meekosha (1999) reminded us that assuming a fixed disability status disadvantages women, who are more likely to have degenerative conditions such as multiple sclerosis and arthritis. Disabled women must "continually renegotiate the relationship between body, self *and* socially constructed disability" (175) in their day-to-day dealings with support systems. One example is chronic fatigue. Wendell (2001) described this as one of the most commonly misunderstood impairments associated with chronic illness. She explained how this particular form of fatigue is qualitatively different from healthy people's experience of fatigue in that it is more debilitating, lasts longer and is less predictable. When she clearly articulates how every action requires energy, including thinking, watching, listening, speaking and eating, the reader cannot help but understand the importance of personal assistance in the form of home support for people who experience this form of impairment, especially when it is recognized that "pushing oneself" can lead to risk of relapse, hospitalization or permanent damage (25). Pain-related disability may also fluctuate over time. Pain impairment is more likely to be reported by women (11.4 percent) than by men (8.8 percent). In fact, young women with disabilities are much more likely to experience pain-related limitations (59.0 percent) than their male counterparts are (42.6 percent) (Cossette and Duclos 2001). Like fatigue, descriptions of the embodied experience of pain can also inform us of the impact of this form of impairment on the need for support when undertaking activities of daily living.

Disputes between national and provincial medical bodies over their level of acceptance of a condition can also cause problems for individual women requesting assistance, especially when the province, responsible for administering home care, publicly denies that a condition such as fibromyalgia, for example, is legitimate. Current procedures for ensuring support discriminate against people, the majority of whom are women, who live with impairments related to conditions that are not always recognized by doctors or easily measured (Council of Canadians with Disabilities 2002). Even when conditions are recognized, they may be considered not sufficiently disabling to warrant service. Through a normalization of disability, society constructs and reinforces the notion that only those with particular impairments are legitimate and worthy of assistance. Professional discourses and texts of home care, including assessment tools and care provision guidelines, frequently operate to disregard women's experience of impairment. Dealing with challenges to their lived realities on an ongoing basis can take a heavy emotional and physical toll on the health of women with disabling chronic illness.

HOME CARE FOR WOMEN WITH DISABILITIES

Women's Need for Care

Disability affects 12.4 percent of the Canadian population residing within households. It affects more women (10.4 percent) than men (9.4 percent) between the ages of 15 and 64 years and more women (42 percent) than men (38 percent) over 65 years of age. Overall, 13.3 percent of women and 11.5 percent of men report a disability (Human Resources Development Canada 2002). In terms of severity, in 2001, at least one in four persons with disabilities (26.9 percent) experienced severe activity limitations and 14.0 percent reported having a very severe disability. A larger proportion of women with disabilities reported a severe level of activity limitation compared to men with disabilities (28.3 percent vs. 25.1 percent). Conversely, men (36.4 percent) were more likely than women (32.2 percent) to report a mild degree of limitation. In total, approximately 1,283,080 women reported having moderate to severe disabilities whereas this level of impairment affected 971,780 men in 2001 (Human Resources Development Canada 2002).

In all age groups, women (12.2 percent) are more likely to have mobility disabilities than men are (8.6 percent). During the working years (15-64 years of age) more women (8.3 percent) than men (6.7 percent) report that less visible pain-related impairment limited their activities. It is important to recognize that people frequently live with multiple impairments – only 18.2 percent of people with disabilities report having a single form of impairment (Statistics Canada 2001b).

It is also worth noting that these statistics exclude the Yukon, Northwest Territories and Nunavut as well as First Nations reserves. The 2000-2001 Canadian Community Health Survey reported that overall rates of disability were significantly higher among Aboriginal peoples than other Canadians (31 percent for those of working age and 53 percent for seniors). Of those with disabilities identified in 1991, the Aboriginal Peoples Survey reported that 45 percent had mobility impairments and 35 percent had disabilities associated with agility (Human Resources Development Canada 2002).

Women and Men with Disabilities Receiving Care

More women with disabilities need support than men with disabilities. However, these women are less likely than their male counterparts to receive the level of care they need. The Participation and Activity Limitation Survey (1991) reported in "Advancing the Inclusion of Persons with Disabilities" that, while 1.1 million women with disabilities needed assistance, only 44 percent of them received all the assistance they needed. In contrast, 700,000 men needed assistance and 50 percent had all they needed (Human Resources Development Canada 2002)

The "Disability Supports: Patterns in Usage and Need among Adult Canadians with Disabilities" document prepared by the Roeher Institute (1995) reported that nearly two million adults with disabilities needed help with one or more everyday activities. Less than half of those (46.3 percent) who needed help received all the assistance they needed and 8 percent needed help but received none. As stated earlier, women are less likely than men to have all the help they need. The same is true for:

- people outside the labour force who consider themselves completely prevented from working because of disability,
- people with low family incomes,
- people who are not receiving disability pensions/benefits,
- people with disability expenses that are not reimbursable by any plan,
- people living in rural communities,
- people with a severe level of disability, and
- older adults.

Major areas of unmet need for help with everyday activities include heavy household chores, regular housework and grocery shopping, although there is also considerable need for help with meal preparation and personal finances. According to the Canadian Community Health Survey (2000-2001) 24 percent of adults with disabilities stated that in the previous 12 months they did not receive all the health care they needed; in the 1994-1995 survey this statistic was 10 percent (Human Resources Development Canada 2002 and Statistics Canada 2001a).

Disability does not exist in isolation. It is important to recognize that women with disabilities experience "interlocking forms of oppression" related to class, race, sexual orientation, (dis)ability status and form of impairment (see Razack 1999:139). These factors affect one another and function to maintain privilege for some and disadvantage for others. For example, women with disabilities experience high rates of unemployment and low or no literacy (Fawcett 1996). Literacy and employment exist within a set of care provision relations that operate to maintain an unjust position for women with disabilities in society. Women who survive on low incomes or who have limited education have greater levels of unmet need (Thomas 1996). Literacy plays a role in enabling people to navigate the health care bureaucracy (Canadian Centre on Disability Studies 2002). Without support to conduct activities of daily living, including engagement with informal and formal educational or job training settings, women with disabilities will continue to experience economic and social disadvantage.

Women who provide care are required to reorganize their lives in order to provide the care that their family members need and women who receive care are forced to reshape personal relationships, such as the mother-daughter relationship, in order to have the care they require. Katz et al. (2000) found that older women with impairments received less informal care (15.7 hours) per week than men with impairments (21.2 hours). The disparity was even greater among married women with disabilities (14.8 hours) and married men with disabilities (26.2 hours). While 44.6 percent of disabled women relied on their children for care, only 22.8 percent of disabled men did. More than 80 percent of these children were daughters, daughters-in-law and granddaughters.

What often goes unrecognized is the fact that many disabled women also provide care to others. The research in this area is limited – probably influenced by the fact that researchers often equate disability with dependency and inadequacy by researchers (see Oliver 1992). However, 20 percent of older disabled women with two or more impairments affecting their daily activities have been found to provide informal care to their spouses. This is a much greater proportion than the disabled male counterparts (8 percent) who provide care to their spouses (Katz et al. 2000).

Disability and Care as Women's Issues

Gender, home care, impairment and disability are interconnected and yet there are, as Marika Morris (2001) pointed out, definite gaps in the literature as it pertains to women with disabilities. There are several ways in which women acquire disabilities more frequently than men. For example, women may acquire long-term impairments through domestic abuse and violence (Meekosha 1999). A number of studies have determined an association between care provision and deteriorating health in women (Canadian Study of Health and Aging 1994). For instance, Keating et al. (1999) found that almost one-third (27.5 percent) of the female unpaid caregivers versus 10.6 percent of male caregivers reported negative health effects resulting from their caregiving role. In fact, a recent study suggested that caregivers experiencing the strain of caregiving have 63 percent higher mortality rates (Schultz and Beach 1999). Gender socialization is not only interwoven with issues of caring, it also plays a direct role in the mechanisms that cause impairment.

Enabling Citizenship for Women with Disabilities

Stereotypical images of citizenship are frequently associated with active and able-bodied white men. These notions need to be challenged. Women who live with disability, for example, are deserving of those conditions that would enable them to contribute fully to their communities, even if their means of engagement are unique.

It is important to consider the political, organizational and interpersonal arrangements that affect the relationships intended to result in the provision of care. It is also critical that women's issues associated with both the provision and acceptance of support be considered. The Roeher Institute and Status of Women Canada (2001) produced a document entitled "Disability-Related Support Arrangements, Policy Options, and Implications for Women's Equality" in which they proposed criteria for equality of well-being between women providing and receiving support, including: promotes self-determination, fosters mutual recognition, encourages respectful interdependence, ensures security, democratizes decision-making processes and promotes citizenship. This report also stated that the promotion of the equality of women's well-being requires that attention be paid to entitlement to supports, assessment procedures, eligibility criteria, access and the framework of benefits. Ultimately this requires "policy and program development that questions the current ideological basis of programs, and that is based on clear and consistent principles of human rights and criteria of equality of well-being" (88).

CAREGIVER–RECEIVER RELATIONSHIP

The inclusion of the perspectives and voices of women who receive home care are essential to an analysis of home care, and issues that affect all women are inextricably linked to broader social and political factors. Globalization and privatization influence home care policies in ways that negatively impact women, both with and without disabilities, who provide and receive care. As a result of these forces, Canadians have witnessed the introduction of policies that shift care to the community without adequate resources. We have also seen a transfer of publicly administered home care services to privately operated and for-profit agencies and privatization that has resulted in the tendering of contracts to those agencies that cut costs by paying staff poorly and prohibiting unions. In addition, we have also witnessed processes that introduced new definitions of "disability" and "home care" in order to reduce the number of people eligible for service and the amount of service provided. All of these have an impact on the level and quality of care, and ultimately affect the provider and the recipient as well as their relationship.

Informal care provision transforms family life. The National Alliance for Care Giving and the American Association of Retired Persons (1997) found that 43 percent of all caregivers report that their caregiving responsibilities have caused them to have less time for other family members than before and to forgo vacations, hobbies and other personal activities (Bookwala and Schultz 2000).

In one focus group, women with disabilities stated that women with children should have enough government-subsidized home support to keep their families together and that their role as "mother" should not be devalued because of the acquisition or existence of impairment. The need for child care or child nurturing assistance has also been recognized within the disability community and yet only a couple of programs offer such a service – for example, the Centre for Independent Living in Toronto and the Centre for Independent Living in Winnipeg. Nurturing support is generally not considered a part of home care and tends only to be provided in extreme circumstances (Masuda 1998). Using home care services to meet child care needs is antithetical to a characterization of women with disabilities as asexual, passive and dependent. In contrast to dominant notions of disability, sexuality and parenting, O'Toole and Doe (2002) presented a discussion of the creative caregiving and innovative independence of disabled parents.

Institutional practices and the discourse of health care management in effect introduce and enforce new meanings for the act of caring, the care provider and those receiving care. Women with impairments in need of assistance have their identity transformed through eligibility assessments that ignore complex, less visible impairments, emphasize inability, and assume passivity. Women informal care providers are expected to provide the majority of care with little or no financial compensation as part of their gendered role. The health care system regulates care, for example, by assessing and requiring informal supports before supplementing care formally within a community context. In these ways loving care becomes transformed into a relation of body maintenance.

Women's negotiation of providing and receiving care is complex. Stress arises in part because of the nature of the demands, and also because of apparent contradictions associated with multiple roles: for example, a young adult woman with a disability continues to depend upon a parent for her basic needs; a child is expected to provide daily personal care to her mother who has a disability; an older woman with memory, fatigue and pain-related impairments continues to provide care to her husband even though she herself is in need of care. These are situations where government-subsidized home care can be introduced to protect full citizenship and opportunity for all women regardless of disability status or stage of life.

Dominant notions of a citizen as a white able-bodied male needs to be challenged, as does the idea that worthy citizens are economically and physically independent taxpayers. In fact, the way we envision how citizenship is enacted – for example, as owning property – needs to be replaced by a much more inclusive and diverse vision. Home care is a prerequisite to full citizenship that is mediated through others – for women with disabilities, their rights, opportunities and responsibilities may be achieved with the provision of formal or informal home support. The rights of the disabled care recipient have been given little attention when the rights of the provider have been emphasized (Walmsley 1993) – consider, for example, the introduction of unions and other forms of safeguards for workers but no equivalent for recipients. As women we need to recognize that these are important considerations for employees and we also need to acknowledge consumers' concern that governments typically find the resources by reducing services to people with disabilities (Mary Ennis, personal communication, 6 April 2003). Administrators who use economic arguments to present provider and receiver needs as mutually exclusive need to be challenged as part of a process of building linkages among disabled and able-bodied women. Canadian policy-makers should address both sets of concerns in recognition of citizenship rights for all women.

The care relationship has been examined by disability scholars and, while some will argue that all people are interdependent (Shakespeare, 2001) others will emphasize that this form of relating is qualitatively distinct. There are important power relations to acknowledge. For example, Twig (2000) described inherently unequal relations within the dynamic of nakedness during bathing when one person is undressed in the presence of another who is fully clothed. In fact, Morris (2001:13) claimed that "the more personal the task the greater the potential for abuse of human rights – and the greater the potential for the 'caregiver' to protect and promote human rights." The care provider's role can be central to achieving full personhood for a woman with a disability. Thus the protection of human rights must be placed at the forefront of our discussions of home care.

One woman with a disability involved in the study described home care and policy-making in the following way: "It's hard enough trying to maintain a life but when you have to rely on other people to help you, you have to be so accommodating, so patient, but that doesn't mean you want to be accommodating and patient to government officials who think that our lives are less valuable" (Krogh 2001a). Members of society often think of patience as a descriptor for the care provider, but within this reciprocal relationship both parties require patience and need to understand the sources of strain that originate outside the relationship. When government-subsidized home care is not provided at sufficient levels, it is not uncommon for recipients to consider this an attack on the value of their contribution as well as their ability and right to contribute economically, socially and politically to their communities (Krogh 2001a).

When women in society are expected to care for others regardless of their own physical, emotional, intellectual and spiritual needs, they become at risk of developing health problems that may interfere directly with the quality of care provision. In fact, as a result of such circumstances, women with disabilities who receive care may be at risk for neglect and abuse. Studies indicate that caregiving responsibilities result in personal and interpersonal loss and that the quality of the caregiver – care recipient relationship deteriorates with increasing care demands (Bookwala and Schultz 2000; Williamson, Shaffer, and Schultz 1998). It has also been found that caregiving wives rated their ongoing relationship with the care recipient to be poorer than did caregiving husbands (Bookwala and Schultz 2000). Among some female providers of care there has been a demonstrated correlation between higher levels of physical and emotional strain (Bookwala and Schultz 1998) as well as greater depressive symptoms in the caregivers (Bookwala, Yee, and Schultz 2000) with perceived higher levels of "behavior problems" in the care recipient. This transformation within the caring relationship could in part be related to the fact that the family becomes engulfed by a health care system that emphasizes, and in fact necessitates, a conceptualization of the care recipient as passive, needy and dependent.

ABUSE AND CARE

Abuse by personal assistance providers is a significant problem especially for women with disabilities. In comparison to able-bodied women, women with disabilities have been found to be more likely to experience abuse by personal assistants and health providers, and they were more likely to experience abuse over a longer time period (Saxton et al. 2001). Sobsey and Doe (1991) also found that having a disability and receiving disability supports played a distinct role in making people vulnerable to abuse. In 44 percent of cases they examined, the abuse took place within a relationship specifically related to the person's disability. In particular, 28 percent of abusers were service providers such as personal care assistants. Less than half of the women reported the abuse because of their fear and their dependence on the abuser.

Abuse or harassment can be linked to multiple sites of discrimination related to, for example, gender, disability or sexual orientation. One woman who relies on home care described the need for peer support for women who receive care and who want to live their lives fully and openly with dignity: "Home support, making people aware of the fact that we have the right to live in our own apartments, we have the right to live our own lives and to live our lives the way we choose, including being gay and living in that lifestyle and all that entails. To have safety around that, to teach people if you're being abused, it's okay to say something. Just because these people care for you doesn't mean they have the right to abuse you" (Krogh et al. 2003).

The form of the abuse must be understood within the unique life context of women with disabilities, including their need for care. For example, women with disabilities may experience neglect and abuse when, after an argument with their care provider, they are left undressed in the shower or on the toilet for long periods of time. Women with disabilities are vulnerable to the effects of a society that devalues them while placing care providers under high levels of personal, physical, emotional and financial stress. In one study women with disabilities identified feeling "mistreated or disrespected by their case managers," "lost in bureaucracy" or being "unfairly rejected for services by agencies" as forms of abuse (Saxton et al. 2001:406). When such abuse and neglect occurs, women with disabilities' ability to participate in daily life activities is compromised as much as their personal emotional and physical health and safety.

High levels of violence, sexual abuse and neglect exist among disabled women (Sobsey and Doe 1991). Given this situation, choice and control over who, when and how care is provided are important considerations for women with disabilities. One woman who grew up in the government system of "care" spoke in her interview with me about the significance of being able to create a safe space for herself by receiving her care through a self-managed care system whereby she personally selected the people hired to provide her personal care: "Home to me means, a little bit different maybe than most people, my home here is the first home I ever had in my life, a space that's mine, a space where I can kind of recoup (sic) from the rest of the world and people that I can bring into my life that I choose to have in my life and feeling safe about it, because I've never had the traditional home life. With that comes working in the framework that I choose to work from as opposed to institutional living or institutional structure and I'm very particular about who I let into my home" (Krogh, 2001a).

CARE AS CONTROL AND SURVEILLANCE

Controlling forces in society construct people with disabilities. Limiting notions of disability are commonly reflected and reinforced by care systems and the interpersonal relationships they encompass (Krogh 2001a). When values that equate disability with dependence become codified within professional discourses, they function as forms of surveillance and discipline (see Foucault 1977) and are thus disabling. In effect, these disabling values can operate ideologically to obscure central issues for people with disabilities, namely social participation and full citizenship (Priestley 1999).

Independence for people with disabilities does not mean doing everything for oneself but it does mean having personal control over how help is provided. A pervasive characteristic of policy-making within the community-based care arena has been the construction of disability as dependency. A unidirectional and causal relationship between impairment and dependency is typically assumed and has been challenged by disability studies scholars such as Michael Oliver (see Oliver 1996). When people with disabilities are assumed to be dependent, they become objects of control.

The central focus should be on issues of citizenship and rights as well as notions of choice and control over care. As Jenny Morris (2001) clearly stated, "Whatever 'care' is – whether it is in the form of formal services, cash payments or personal relationships – if it does not enable people 'to state an opinion,' 'to participate in decisions which affect their lives' and 'to share fully in the social life of their community' then it will be unethical" (15). She concludes that society is in need of an ethic of care based on the principle that to deny the human rights of our fellow human beings is to undermine our own humanity. Home care provision should recognize that all people, regardless of the nature of their impairment, have the capacity to express preferences.

Even when services are supplied directly to the person with a disability, they are frequently not delivered in a way that enables people with disabilities to have control over their activities of daily living or community participation (Barnes et al. 1999). Disabled researchers have pointed out their concern that care providers are viewed to be in need of resources and support – it is implied that they are in a position to speak on behalf of those who require care (Morris, 1993). Given these restrictions, community care has been described as "the most exploitative of all forms of so-called care delivered in our society today for it exploits both the person providing and receiving care and these are most likely to be women rather than men. It ruins relationships between people and results in thwarted life opportunities on both sides of the caring equation" (Brisenden 1989:10).

The focus of care administration is not on how care can be provided to support individuals in meeting their self-identified needs within a framework of their immediate and longer term life priorities, but on monitoring what type of care service is provided – when, where, by whom and at what level. Care management procedures and instruments function to control expenditures (Browne 2000). They are also products of a society that constructs and expects people with disabilities to be dependent, passive and eternally grateful (see, for example, Linton 1998 for a discussion of this construction of disability). Morgan's (1995) study results, based on a social service survey of 26,000 households, found that only 7 percent of the households had long-term sick or disabled persons within them. Of these households, only 2 percent reported any use of social services, challenging dominant notions of people with disabilities as a drain on the system.

Female bodies are more likely to be the objects of regulation and surveillance by a patriarchal state (Meekosha 1999). Disabled women, in greater numbers than disabled men, have been incarcerated in prisons, hospitals, nursing homes and a multitude of institutions (Australian Institute of Health and Welfare 1993). Women are also over-represented as social service recipients (Ferguson 2000). When women with disabilities attempt to access services such as government-subsidized home care, they must be expected to give up what Orme (2001) referred to as their right to freedom from interference and their right not to reveal details of their personal life.

In addition, people with disabilities effectively have their everyday lives dominated by a health care management system of assessment and surveillance that does not offer adequate access to appeal procedures or independent confidential complaint mechanisms. The Council of Canadians with Disabilities (CCD) stated that the most common reason why people with impairments seek medical appointments is to have their disability certified in order to receive benefits. CCD seriously questioned whether this form of surveillance is the best use of Canada's health resources (Council of Canadians with Disabilities 2002:47). In a national study conducted by the DisAbled Women's Network (Masuda 1998) one participant described control in relation to a woman with a mental health disability who was cut off from benefits because she had not seen her doctor regularly. She stated, "You are required to make regular visits to your doctor, whether or not you need it, just to reaffirm that you are still disabled" (4). In general, the women with disabilities described how it was increasingly difficult to qualify for disability benefits. A woman in Nova Scotia stated that, "It seems there is a fear that people may be pretending to be disabled and someone may actually get benefits that they don't deserve. When applying for benefits, women with mental health disabilities are always turned down unless they have strong advocacy support" (4). Similar circumstances exist for people who rely on benefits, including home care service associated with employee benefits programs after they acquire a long-term impairment.

Silencing the "Other"

Cultural imperialism involves the universalization of a dominant group's experience and culture resulting in its establishment as the norm (Bourdieu and Passeron 1977; Young 1990). Through this process people with disabilities are simultaneously made invisible through cultural norms and identified as visibly different, reinforced by stereotypes. Ultimately these function to create and isolate the "other." Proctor (2001) offers an important piece of work in which older people with memory impairments come to see themselves as unworthy of even an explanation of their care. One participant in Proctor's study stated, "I should have been given an explanation. Well, I shouldn't. They haven't got time to give everyone explanations" (369). This example illustrates how dominant norms or notions related to being a passive and grateful recipient of care can become internalized by women with disabilities. It also represents a form of symbolic violence (Bourdieu 1985).

To be successful in applying for home care, a person with a disability must often internalize assessment standards, clearly articulating and demonstrating her dependency. While this process can be viewed as an act of legitimating administrative surveillance (see Foucault 1977) it is also often experienced, at the immediate individual level, as a necessary act for survival. Emphasizing dependency creates an internal discord for many people who live with impairments as it runs counter to many individuals' goals to live and be portrayed as self-determining and independent or interdependent. The direct funding programs represent one way that notions of need for care and self-direction have attempted to be reconciled, but the outcome has been one of mixed results.

SELF-DIRECTED CARE

Self-managed care programs are under provincial jurisdiction – and therefore differ among the provinces in terms of administrative structures and eligibility criteria (Keefe and Fancey 1998) – and are intended to increase choice and control by enabling care recipients to purchase and manage their own home care. Within this model, the consumer receives funds directly from the government or via a government-appointed nonprofit agency such as an Independent Living Resource Centre. By way of a contract, the person with long-term impairments who requires assistance agrees to act as the employer and use the funds for purchasing services. In this way, the government attempts to no longer be responsible for employer responsibilities such as those associated with labour standards.

These programs have tremendous potential because of the increased levels of choice, control and independence. However, in reality, there are several challenges that limit the realization of these ideals. The consumer is expected to assume the roles of personnel manager, financial administrator and staff trainer without compensation. While it is clear that such a system saves money, it is frustrating for consumers who are not provided with enough funds to ensure reliable and quality care. Employees must often be willing to work at a lower wage with fewer benefits compared to most agency- or government-administered care. As the coordinator of the Home Support Action Group in Victoria, B.C. explained, "the fundamental flaw of these programs is that they are set up so that the potential for self-determination is the very last consideration" (Gordon Argyle, personal communication, 7 April 2003).

As stated previously, people who receive services may internalize the dominant societal norms reflected in home care policy, administration and service. Interestingly, there has been some research on how people who use direct funding come to view themselves in relation to their impairment and society. Those who received services delivered through traditional means tended to view their own impairment and its effects on mobility as the cause of their problems. In contrast, those people who directed their own care were more likely to view barriers outside of the body in locations such as physical architecture and societal attitudes (Kvetoslava 1999). This shift corresponds with a move away from an internalization of an individualized medical model of disability to one that more holistically portrays disability within a socio-political context.

The personal control that can be associated with self-directed care provides a sense of safety for some women with disabilities. One female participant stated: "I fought so hard to get here, so hard to have independence and so hard to have safety.... If you give me the control, I have an element of safety but if somebody else has that control, I would be devastated" (Krogh 2001a).

Some research indicated that the majority of people with disabilities wish to have the option of receiving their care through a self-directed program rather than administered through an agency (Kestenbaum 1992). This research also found that such programs produce increased flexibility in terms of what type of services are provided and when. They are frequently perceived as empowering because recipients have a greater say in developing and monitoring their own support system and in leading their lives as they choose (Kestenbaum 1993a, 1993b; Morris 1993). From the funder's perspective, it has been viewed as a less costly option than government-administered community-based care or residential services (Hollander et al. 1994).

The role of disability organizations in providing peer support to those using self-directed care is critical given that oppression and exclusion result in fewer opportunities for people with disabilities to develop their skills as managers. A central purpose of the care, i.e., exercising citizenship rights for community participation, needs to be acknowledged. Without addressing these concerns, direct funding only provides women and men with disabilities with an opportunity to become more directly involved in a system that oppresses them.

Flexibility in relation to the nature and site of all home care service is required regardless of the system of administration. Home care, when it works well, can enable many people with disabilities to define themselves and their lifestyles in ways that might counter dominant societal norms. Referring to cuts in services and service options, one participant stated, "It will affect our freedom, our level of independence and what we classify as independence – being stuck back in boxes as opposed to being able to choose, people imposing values and beliefs ... of how it should be" (Krogh 2001a).

However, self-determination is only possible when adequate levels of resources are provided. As Priestley (1999) contended, those who do not have adequate levels of resources are placed in a position of "self-regulation and surveillance, forced to impose upon themselves the values of a welfare system which prioritizes treatment over social integration and participatory citizenship" (670).

ECONOMICS AND EFFICIENCY

Economics

Many studies have calculated the costs of care and projected economic comparisons between institutional and community-based care. For example, the total home care (all forms of home care including post-acute care) spending in Canada was $3.4 billion in the 2000-2001 fiscal year. Of this amount, about

$0.7 billion (20 percent) came from private sources and the remaining $2.7 billion (80 percent) from public sources (Coyte 2000). The rhetoric during the past decade espoused a need to manage uncontrolled health care spending. However, such concerns arose at the same time that those costs began to stabilize as a share of the Gross Domestic Product (GDP) (Evans 1993) and by the mid-1990s governments at all levels had contained health care costs (Rachlis and Kushner 1994).

Costs and impacts of home care versus institutional care have been investigated in a series of fifteen substudies coordinated by Neena Chappell and Marcus Hollander. One of these studies (Hollander et al. 2002) for example, included 580 individuals over 65 years of age in B.C. and Manitoba who require home or institutional care. It was found that home care costs to government were on average approximately 40-50 percent of residential care costs. Interestingly, it was found that recipients of home care services and informal caregivers contributed approximately half of the care costs of the community clients and about one-third of the care costs of facility clients. This demonstrates how the shift away from hospital-based care to community-based care has been used to redirect and reduce costs for governments. They conclude their study with the question, "Is it reasonable for government to pay fully for short-term curative care provided by physicians and hospitals but not pay the same proportion for people with ongoing care needs?" (3).

Efficiency

As an ideology, efficiency is used to justify the erosion of the Canadian health care system (Burke 2000). Underlying the use of efficiency as a measure of public policy worth, is the debate between the role of the state versus the role of the market. It also reflects an appreciation of independent rather than collective or interdependent notions of rights and responsibilities (Tuohy 1992). This has direct implications for people with disabilities who wish to live independently or interdependently. Canadian politics increasingly favours the market, decentralization and individualism, which will continue to have a negative impact on women who provide and receive informal and formal care.

Efficiency is part of an atomizing, isolating and individualizing discourse and it operates to degrade social capital in the form of social organization, including networks, norms and trust (Putnam 1993). Such social capital is crucial to social coordination and the organization of forms of resistance to change. Efficiency can thus be used to reduce social and political participation of citizens. Burke (2000) argued that ultimately the principles of quality, equity and universality are being sacrificed to the narrow concerns of efficiency. As illustrated elsewhere in this chapter, this has been witnessed in relation to home care and, specifically, women.

Numerous researchers have pointed out that economic arguments for home care do not consider all of the true costs of care, particularly as they relate to the impacts upon women caregivers (Fast et al. 1999). Disabled people are directed to rely largely on informal care providers, charities and nonprofit organizations for the support they need (Krogh et al. 2003; Krogh 2001a). For people with disabilities, relying on unskilled community volunteers to provide home care through charities is problematic for many reasons. Not least, it requires people with disabilities to assume the degrading role of objects of pity in order to get what they need. In response to the final recommendations report of the Romanow Commission on the Future of Health Care in Canada, the Council of Canadians with Disabilities (CCD) wrote to the Federal Minister of Health commending the recommended efforts to begin to address the home support needs of people with mental health disabilities. The Council also clearly stated their overall concerns about the low priority given to home support for people with all forms of impairment. CCD wrote, "[i]t is a grave disservice to a host of persons with disabilities across Canada that Mr. Romanow has decided that their home support needs are not on a par to those of other populations. It is especially alarming that Mr. Romanow has decided that our citizenship rights are too expensive to be maintained, therefore our needs are not a priority worthy of being addressed in a timely and appropriate fashion" (Council of Canadians with Disabilities, 22 January 2003).

When people with disabilities are required to approach charities for basic services such as baths, they are thus invited to participate in their own oppression by constructing themselves in terms of their personal failings and as objects of pity, rather than in terms of their abilities and valuable contributions to society, or as citizens deserving of a basic right to self-determination (Krogh et al. 2003). The option of going to a consumer-directed organization for peer support or care management training is seriously impeded when these nonprofit community organizations have their core funding continually reduced or threatened (Boyce et al. 1999). Michael Hall and Paul Reed (1998) concluded that the second social net of voluntary organizations is too small and vulnerable to handle what governments expect of them when they cut funding to such organizations and their programs.

Efficiency necessitates the construction of care recipients as passive and dependent and does not make room for either notions of collaborative engagement in tasks, or consumer prioritization of activities to support social and economic participation in society from the perspective of the person receiving home care. A self-determined process can take time – a person with an impairment affecting learning or cognition may need concepts presented in plain language supplemented with drawings, and if socialized to be passive, she may need access to peer support to review her options before making a decision. A person receiving information related to such a decision from a woman using an augmentative and alternative communication system will need to wait to receive information as each symbol or letter is pointed to in sequence.

Efficiency discourse poses several problems for people with disabilities. In terms of service and accomplishment of home care-related tasks, people with disabilities often accomplish their tasks differently from able-bodied people. For many it is centrally important that they participate as much as possible in directing and engaging in their activities of daily living, including services provided through home care, even if it takes longer. A service system that emphasizes time is inherently problematic, especially when this is done at the expense of self-determination and dignity for people who live with impairments.

The needs and desires of people with disabilities become secondary to the efficiency of the system. Referring to a reorganization of her home support after a home care contract tendering process in her region, an interviewee stated: "When they changed the system around, they changed those hours on me too which meant that I had to retrain my body to go to the bathroom at a slightly different timeframe.... It took a while, and the stress of it was just [incredible], because I didn't know if I could do it. I had had those hours for about 14 years and overnight ... like forget it. (Krogh 2001a).

HOME CARE AND FULL CITIZENSHIP

Disability and Citizenship

While there seems to be a general acknowledgement that people with disabilities in Canada need and deserve supports, many of the existing home care policies do not reflect this notion. For example, Canadian government reports such as "In Unison: A Canadian Approach to Disability Issues," reflect the notion that people with disabilities should receive support in their efforts to be active in their communities and society (Government of Canada 2000). However, people with disabilities in Canada clearly struggle to receive the home support they need (British Columbia Coalition of People with Disabilities, 2000). A woman who requires home support proposed some questions for policy-makers to consider, based on her own life experience: "How would you feel if you were stuck in bed and couldn't get out? And all you could do was not get out the door, not get up to turn on the radio or you know, go to the fridge and get yourself a drink whenever you wanted to, even in your own home, that wouldn't be living – to live in your own bed is no life at all" (Krogh 2001a).

Home care for people with disabilities is a sociopolitical issue, not an individual medical problem. Conceptualizing home support in terms of medical procedures solely within the home acts to divert attention away from the rights for citizenship and the role of society in creating or addressing social, economic and political issues that impose restrictions. The reification of social problems into individual medical concerns has been discussed in both feminist health literature (Pirie 1988; Wuest 1993) and disability studies literature (Morris 1993). The social model of disability with a recognition of the value of phenomenological descriptions of embodied experience form a valuable basis for understanding the significance of home support in the lives of women with disabilities.

The ideologies of "caring" and "efficiency" in combination with the dominance of the individualistic medical model of disability within home care have operated to undermine the citizenship and civil rights of disabled people. Women with disabilities experience systemic discrimination in education, employment and health care. State-assured citizenship protections and rights appear to have little application in the lives of many of these women. Feminist disability researcher Jenny Morris (2001) concluded that, "in many situations the human and civil rights of disabled people cannot be promoted without particular action being taken, resources being made available, which would give us equal access. Specific entitlements (that is, different treatment) are necessary for equal access" (11).

After an extensive community consultation process, Prince Edward Island has introduced a disability-supports program in which individual recipients are allowed choice in determining the type of support they need in order to achieve their personal goals. Since the introduction of the program, this approach has supported increasing numbers of people in returning to or entering the workforce (Brian Bertelsen, Coordinator of Disability Supports and Services for Prince Edward Island, personal communication, 25 January 2003). However, it is important to note that monthly financial caps on services present significant barriers to achieving personal goals, including community living for those individuals who require relatively high levels of care.

People with disabilities receiving home support have had to fight to receive and maintain levels and types of support as new, more restrictive guidelines are introduced related to the type of services provided. For example, some regions have removed meal preparation or social participation supports (Health Canada 1999). Other regions no longer include housekeeping, reflecting a definition of health and home support that no longer includes household hygiene (Krogh et al. 2003; Krogh 2001a). Such a trend is of particular concern to women who live with compromised immune systems. Supports located outside of the home that facilitate community participation are increasingly being considered unnecessary. New and future users of home care are at particular risk of never receiving the level of care they need to enable them to engage in society as full citizens (Roeher Institute and Status of Women Canada 2001).

Home care is required by many disabled people for access to their communities and a full range of life opportunities. Independent living principles include flexibility, choice and control as well as access to peer support. As Morris (1993) pointed out, when the philosophy and aims associated with the independent living movement are neither understood nor accepted, community care policy initiatives only result in institutionalization within the community. Flexibility, choice and control within home and community settings are not only important social determinants of health, their presence or absence constitutes the distinction between institutional and community living (Priestley 1998, 1999). Choice in relation to the care provider has been associated with health outcomes, but studies have generally not examined the negative impact of having care imposed in ways that offer limited choice to the care receiver. For women with disabilities, choice might be in the form of: the administration of care (direct care, agency care, supported living or institutional care); the nature of the tasks involved (personal hygiene, house cleaning, accompanying a person doing their shopping, assisting a person with the physical act of organizing course papers while studying for an exam); or the organization of the delivery of care (sequence, priority activities, location).

Women, Disability and Citizenship

Women with disabilities are frequently assumed to be dependent, passive and needy, rather than interdependent and active contributors to their communities. Their exclusion from citizenship discussions may be further complicated when the nature of their contributions does not conform to society's expectations. Thus, as mentioned earlier, society's images of citizenship omit disability by reflecting and perpetuating hegemonic notions of normalcy (Meekosha and Dowse 1997). Disability challenges our use of simple binaries such as rights versus duties within citizenship debates because the assumption is that these are guided by people with able bodies who are free to accept assistance or not.

Within a feminist critique of citizenship, women need to become aware of those forms of citizenship that for some necessitate the categorization of women with disabilities as objects of caring work (Meekosha and Dowse 1997). We also need to recognize our interconnectedness within communities and focus on the development of strategies that acknowledge a full range of experiences and foster effective participation for all women.

One disabled woman in the study described the interpersonal relationship that enables citizenship through the provision of home support in the following way:

> Everything that we want to do outside our own home and to be up and about in your own home, to have people in, you need home care in order to do that and the quality of home care is important because for a younger disabled adult, you need a person that is flexible and understands that you don't just live for a person walking into your house to get you up, get you dressed, give you a bath, you have a life outside your apartment and therefore they are just a small part of your life ... but in another instance they are also the most important part of your life because you cannot do anything else if you can't get out of bed. (Krogh and the Home Support Action Group 2000)

Citizenship rights are located in both social and political arenas. Nira Yuval-Davis (1997) explained that, without "enabling" social conditions, political rights are vacuous and at the same time, citizenship rights without obligations also construct people as passive and dependent. She concluded that, "the most important duty of citizens, therefore, is to exercise their political right and to participate in the determination of their collectivities', states', and societies' trajectories" (21-22).

Citizenship rights must be extended to provide opportunities for engagement to people with disabilities in the development of home care policy, programs, program evaluation, eligibility criteria, assessment tools and procedures. Most importantly, all home care programs must incorporate an accessible appeal mechanism that includes representation from organizations that are consumer-directed: i.e., led by persons with disabilities, including disabled women's organizations. The importance of an arm's-length relationship of such an appeal board has been emphasized (Community Living Transition Steering

Committee 2002). Particular attention should be paid to the various forms of impairment, gender issues and the need for peer support and self-determination.

The full implications of citizenship need to be acknowledged by the women providing and receiving care, within the context of their relationship. Canada needs a set of national home care standards in order to establish expectations for the provinces.

THE NEED FOR A NATIONAL STANDARD

Administration of home care is a provincial responsibility and several studies have documented that, without a national standard, there are significant differences among the provinces in terms of eligibility criteria, user fees and range of service (see Health Canada 1999). Variations also exist in terms of how publicly funded home care is delivered: direct provision by public employees, competitive tendering by private agencies, partnership between government and nonprofit providers, and self-managed care (Campbell et al. 2002).

The reworking of eligibility criteria appears to be designed to create ineligibility to reduce costs rather than to facilitate the exercising of rights. This has been seen, for example, through the redefining of terms used to regulate home care service including: disability, eligibility criteria and types of services. Consequently, Canadians who live with long-term impairments are at increasing risk of being arbitrarily reassessed as eligible for less or no care. Reassessment can be introduced in waves through particular regions or it can be initiated by such factors as an individual's move to a new region. This is a mobility rights issue because a move to a new region necessarily involves a reassessment. The Charter of Rights and Freedoms is intended for all Canadians but the freedom of mobility rights as articulated by section 6(2)(a) which states that "every citizen of Canada and every person who has the status of a permanent resident of Canada has the right to move to and take up residence in any province" does not seem to apply to Canadians who rely on government-subsidized home care. People with disabilities who require home support are not free to move from one province to another, nor are they necessarily free to move within their own province. The Council of Canadians with Disabilities now advises people with disabilities requiring home care to think very carefully before moving to a new region, province or territory because the reassessment that such a move triggers is likely to result in fewer hours of home care (Laurie Beachell, personal communication, 24 January 2003).

One report entitled "Without Foundation" (Pollak and Cohen 2000) reviewed health care in B.C. and provided alerts to other regions in Canada undergoing health care restructuring. The authors concluded that inadequate funding has created a growing gap between health needs and the public services available. They went on to state that, rather than focusing on prevention and early intervention, health care services have become increasingly crisis-oriented. They described the cuts to home support in B.C. as "drastic" and claim that they have created "an explosion of problems for patients, family members, care providers and health administrators" (6). Specifically, they referred to declining health due to poor nutrition, stress and isolation; hospitalization; higher rates of injury among workers; and the denial of people's basic human right to live at home and participate in their community.

Social participation is critical to the efforts of all people with disabilities to achieve full citizenship. Yet some provinces do not consider this a legitimate rationale for accessing home care and other services. Disabled people will probably be kept alive in their rooms but will not be enabled to venture beyond the four walls of their bedrooms or homes (Krogh 2001a; Krogh and the Home Support Action Group 2000). Social participation supports health. As one woman with a disability who relies on home care stated, "the more we're involved in our community, the healthier we are – with our [physical] health, our mental health" (Krogh 2001a).

It is well recognized that people with disabilities experience a number of "disincentives" to work, including the cost of technology and the risks associated with losing medical coverage. Increasingly, women with disabilities who are offered employment must further assess the costs of becoming employed given that, in many provinces, they will be expected to pay user fees for their own home care once they start earning an income. The application of user fees and other factors considered in determining the amount of payment required – e.g. assets or cash in the bank – varies among the provinces and territories.

The disability community has been calling for National Standards for Home Care for several years (Council of Canadians with Disabilities 2002). Given the historical conflict between the federal and provincial governments, provinces appear unable to commit to a policy of consistent, quality standards of home care for disabled people. At this time, federal leadership is required to assure citizenship rights for all Canadians. Given the various service delivery methods, e.g., private, nonprofit, government and self-directed administration, it is unlikely that a single model can be mandated within all regions. A set of national principles or standards for home support put forward by the federal government can be achieved through a variety of means by provinces in order to qualify for federal dollars (Campbell et al. 2002). Cost-sharing between provincial and federal governments, as well as across those ministries responsible for health, employment, education and social services could also be considered.

CONCLUDING COMMENTS

Canada requires a set of national home care standards that explicitly recognize the role of home support as a necessary service that mediates citizenship. A national standard would eliminate significant variations that currently exist among provinces and territories, and would thus not only assure a precondition for equal opportunities for citizen participation, but also represent a move to protect mobility rights as outlined in section 6(2)(a) and equality rights under section 15 of the *Charter of Rights and Freedoms* for people with disabilities. Modes of delivery could vary as long as sufficient funds are provided to deliver quality home care.

A direct-funding program option must be made available in all provinces and territories. It is crucial that this method of care delivery be accompanied by sufficient resources for both the service and consumer-directed organizations that can provide subcontracted assistance, training and peer support. All regions of Canada need to have an impartial appeal mechanism that includes guiding principles related to promoting citizenship and equal opportunity as well as certain restrictions to limit the influence of economics in decision-making. Flexible service in terms of the nature of tasks that are performed, and where and how they are organized within the context of the disabled woman's life is essential. National standards should include a range of services including meal preparation and house cleaning that are frequently required, yet increasingly being eliminated because they are not seen as medically necessary.

Definitions of disability, home support and citizenship reflected in and reinforced through home support policy must be re-examined and challenged. In particular, the individualistic medical definition of disability needs to be replaced by a sociopolitical definition of disability that acknowledges phenomenological embodied and situated expertise; the notion of home support as merely a medical service needs to be greatly expanded to acknowledge that it is also a facilitator of citizen participation; and the idea must be discarded that those who live interdependently rather than independently are passive and less worthy members of society.

Home care and disability are gendered issues. For example, care recipients and providers are most likely to be women; poor working and living conditions for paid and unpaid care providers lead to increasing numbers of women becoming disabled through long-term injuries or the aggravation of a chronic condition; and disabled women must negotiate their various socially influenced roles, including parent and caregiver. Existing policies and programs differentially disadvantage women with disabilities in comparison to men with disabilities. In addition, they particularly discriminate against women with certain forms of impairments – for example, those related to nonvisible chronic illness, developmental disability and mental health impairment as well as women who experience interlocking forms of discrimination related to, for instance, race, ethnicity, sexual orientation, poverty or literacy. Programs must reflect a commitment to reduce the systemic social, economic and political discrimination based on gender, class, race, ethnicity and sexual orientation that women with disabilities experience. Disabled women who rely on home support deserve to be provided with assurances of safety and respect in ways that recognize their identities, expertise, priorities and personhood. These points must be considered in policy-making, program design and the creation of meaningful and accessible opportunities for women with disabilities to participate in policy-making, program design, implementation, evaluation and appeal procedures.

Home care is ultimately about voice. When home care does not work well, women with disabilities live in isolation from their communities and in fear of arbitrary decisions made about eligibility for supports. Within Canadian society, we have seen a number of developments, such as more accessible municipal transit, that are intended to facilitate engagement in society for people with disabilities, but without home supports, many people with disabilities cannot get out of bed to access such services. Inadequate levels of home support and a limited choice about the nature of its provision in effect act to institutionalize people within the confines of their own homes. It is necessary to reconsider political processes and home support administrative systems and the values that underlie them in order to create opportunities for people, especially women with disabilities, from a range of social locations. Representatives from disabled women's organizations, ethnocultural disability organizations and cross-disability organizations must play a role in policy design, program implementation and evaluation and serve on appeal committees.

Finally, we must recognize that issues affecting all women are inextricably linked whether we consider care providers, care recipients or both. Efforts to improve home support policy, programs and services for care recipients must be advocated for alongside improved working conditions for women who provide the majority of formal and informal care. Together we can work to improve the social, political and economic circumstances that directly influence the quality of the care relationship.

Disability activists have made it clear that home care for people with disabilities should be considered a right not a luxury (British Columbia Coalition of People with Disabilities 2000; Council of Canadians with Disabilities 2002). The essence of home support as an essential component of life was made vivid when one woman with a disability in the study stated: "I can't plan ahead because tomorrow morning, they might cut my hours back … so what I've been doing for the last whatever number of years that I've been having these hours [threatened is] … I'm living day to day … and how would that impact your life if you couldn't plan for next week or next month or the summer? I mean, people don't plan day to day, they make a plan for the future. At this moment, I don't have any plans for the future because I don't know what the future will bring. If I can't get out of bed, there's no use planning anything" (Krogh 2001a).

The author would like to acknowledge personnel support and research grants from the Canadian Institutes of Health Research and the Social Sciences and Humanities Research Council.

References

Australian Institute of Health and Welfare. (1993). *Australia's Welfare 1993: Services and Assistance.* Canberra: Australian Government Publishing Service.

Barnes, C., G. Mercer, and T. Shakespeare. (1999). *Exploring Disability: A Sociological Introduction.* Malden, MA: Blackwell.

Bookwala, J., J.L. Yee and R. Schultz. (2000). "Caregiving and Detrimental Mental and Physical Health Outcomes," p. 93-131 in D.M. Williamson, P.A. Parmelee and D.R. Shaffer (eds.), *Physical Illness and Depression in Older Adults: A Handbook of Theory, Research and Practice.* New York: Plenum.

Bookwala, J. and R. Schultz. (1998). "The Role of Neuroticism and Mastery in Spouse Caregivers' Assessment of and Response to a Contextual Stressor." *Journal of Gerontology: Psychological Sciences,* 53B, 155-164.

———— (2000). "A Comparison of Primary Stressors, Secondary Stressors, and Depressive Symptoms Between Elderly Caregiving Husbands and Wives: The Caregiver Health Effects Study." *Psychology and Aging, 15,* 607-616.

Bourdieu, P. (1985). *Outline of a Theory of Practice.* Cambridge, UK: Cambridge University Press. (Original work published in 1972 as *Esquisse d'une theorie de la pratique*).

Bourdieu, P. and J.C. Passeron. (1977). *Reproduction in Education, Society and Culture.* Beverly Hills, CA: Sage.

Boyce, W., K. Krogh, J. Kaufert, J. Hall, C. La France and H. Enns. (1999, May). "How Consumer Organizations of People With Disabilities are Responding to Social, Economic and Political Change," p. 151-156 in proceedings from conference entitled *Research to Action: Working Together for the Integration of Canadians With Disabilities.* Halifax, Nova Scotia.

Brisenden, S. (1989). *A Charter for Personal Care* (Progress 16). London: The Disablement Income Group.

British Columbia Coalition of People with Disabilities. (2000, July/August). "Home Support: The Quiet Crisis" [Special issue], *Transitions Magazine.* Vancouver, British Columbia.

Browne, P.L. (2000). *Unsafe Practices: Restructuring and Privatization in Ontario Health Care.* Ottawa, Ontario: Canadian Centre for Policy Alternatives.

Burke, M. (2000). "Efficiency and the Erosion of Health Care in Canada," p. 178-193 in M. Burke, C. Mooers and J. Shields (eds.), *Restructuring and Resistance: Canadian Public Policy in an Age of Global Capitalism.* Halifax, Nova Scotia: Fernwood.

Campbell, B., C. Blouin, J. Foster, R. Labonte, J. Lexchin, M. Sanger, S. Shrybman and S. Sinclair. (2002). *Putting Health First: Canadian Health Care Reform, Trade Treaties and Foreign Policy.* Ottawa, Ontario: Canadian Centre for Policy Alternatives.

Canadian Centre on Disability Studies. (2002). *Report of a Study of the Accessibility of Adult Literacy Programs for Individuals with Disabilities in Manitoba.* Winnipeg, MB.

Canadian Study of Health and Aging. (1994). "Patterns of Caring for People with Dementia in Canada." *Canadian Journal on Aging, 13,* 470-487.

Clare, E. (1999). *Exile and Pride: Disability, Queerness and Liberation.* Cambridge, MA: South End Press.

Community Living Transition Steering Committee. (2002). *Recommendations Report, Ministry of Children and Family Development, BC.* Retrieved 6 May 2003, from http://www.cltsc.bc.ca/Final_Report.htm

Cossette, L. and E. Duclos. (2001). *A Profile of Disability in Canada, 2001* (Report from Statistics Canada, Housing, Family and Social Statistics Division). Ottawa, Ontario: Government of Canada.

Council of Canadians with Disabilities. (2002). *Consumers with Disabilities Speak Out on Health Issues* (Submission to the Romanow Commission on the Future of Health Care in Canada). Winnipeg, Manitoba.

———— (2003, January 22). *Letter to Federal Minister of Health Anne McLellan.* Winnipeg, Manitoba.

Coyte, P. (2000). "Home Care in Canada: Passing the Buck." *Canadian Journal of Nursing Research, 33*(2), 11-25.

Evans, R.G. (1993, July-August). "Health Care Reform: The Issue From Hell." *Policy Options, 14.*

Fast, J., G.M. Williamson and N. Keating. (1999). "The Hidden Costs of Informal Elder Care." *Journal of Family and Economic Issues, 20*, 301-326.

Fawcett, G. (1996). *Living with Disability in Canada: An Economic Portrait.* Ottawa: Human Resources Development Canada, Office for Disability Issues.

Ferguson, S. (2000). "Beyond the Welfare State? Left Feminism and Global Capitalist Restructuring," p. 276-286 in M. Burke, C. Mooers and J. Shields (eds.), *Restructuring and Resistance: Canadian Public Policy in an Age of Global Capitalism.* Halifax, Nova Scotia: Fernwood.

Foucault, M. (1973). *The Birth of the Clinic: An Archaeology of Medical Perception* (A.M.S. Smith, trans.). New York: Vintage Books. (Originally published 1963 as *Naissance de la Clinique.*)

———— (1977). *Discipline and Punish: The Birth of the Prison* (A. Sheridan, trans.). New York: Random House. (Originally published 1975 as *Surveiller et Punir: Naissance de la Prison.*)

Government of Canada. (2000). *In Unison: People with Disabilities in Canada.* Retrieved 6 May 2003, from Human Resources Development Canada Web site: http://socialunion.gc.ca/In_Unison2000

Hall, M. and P. Reed. (1998). "Shifting the Burden: How Much can Government Download to the Non-profit Sector?" *Canadian Public Administration, 41(1), 1-20.*

Health Canada. (1999, June). *Provincial and Territorial Home Care Programs: A Synthesis for Canada.* Retrieved 6 May 2003, from Health Canada Web site: http://www.hc-sc.gc.ca

Hollander, M.J.N. Chappell, B. Havens, C. McWilliam and J.A. Miller. (2002). *Research Report for Substudy 5: Study of the Costs and Outcomes of Home Care and Residential Long-term Care Services* (Report for the Health Transitions Fund). Victoria, BC: University of Victoria and Hollander Analytic Services.

Hooyman, N.R. and J.G. Gonyea. (1999). "A Feminist Model of Family Care: Practice and Policy Directions." *Journal of Women and Aging, 11,* 149-169.

Human Resources Development Canada. (2002). *Advancing the Inclusion of Persons with Disabilities.* Ottawa: Government of Canada. Retrieved 6 May 2003, from http://www.hrdc-drhc.gc.ca/hrib/sdd-dds/odi/documents/AIPD/fdr000.shtml

Humphrey, J.C. (2000). "Researching Disability Politics, or, Some Problems with the Social Model in Practice." *Disability and Society,* 15(1), 63-85.

Katz, S.J., M. Kabeto and K.M. Langa. (2000). "Gender Disparities in the Receipt of Home Care for Elderly People with Disability in the United States." *Journal of the American Medical Association,* 284, 3022-3027.

Keating, N., J. Fast, J. Frederick, K. Cranswick and C. Perrier. (1999). *Eldercare in Canada: Context, Content and Consequences.* Ottawa, Ontario: Statistics Canada.

Keefe, J.M. and P.J. Fancey. (1998). *Financial Compensation Versus Community Supports: An Analysis of the Effects on Caregivers and Care Receivers* (Final report for Health Canada). Halifax, Nova Scotia: Mount Saint Vincent University, Department of Gerontology.

Kestenbaum, A. (1992). *Cash for Care.* Nottingham, UK: Independent Living Fund.

———— (1993a). *Taking Care in the Market: A Study of Agency Homecare.* London, UK: Royal Association for Disability and Rehabilitation and The Disablement Income Group.

———— (1993b). *Making Community Care a Reality: The Independent Living Fund 1988-1993.* London, UK: Royal Association for Disability and Rehabilitation and The Disablement Income Group.

Kitwood, T. and K. Bredin. (1992). "A New Approach to the Evaluation of Dementia Care." *Journal of Advances in Health and Nursing Care, 1*(5), 41-60.

Krogh, K. (2001a, April). *Beyond Four Walls: Impact of Home Support on Work, Health and Citizenship of People with Disabilities* (Multimedia research report distributed at the World Health Organization's Rethinking Care from the Perspectives of People with Disabilities: A Global Congress). Retrieved 6 May 2003, from http://www.ryerson.ca/~kkrogh

———— (2001b, June). *Video Action Research: Possibilities as an Emancipatory Research Methodology and Reflections on a Health Policy Study for People with Disabilities.* Paper presented at the conference of the Society of Disability Studies, Winnipeg, Manitoba.

Krogh, K. and the Home Support Action Group. (2000). *Beyond Four Walls: Impact of Home Support on Health, Work and Citizenship for People with Disabilities* (Research-based video resulting from study funded by the Social Sciences and Humanities Research Council). Victoria, British Columbia: University of Victoria, Faculty of Human and Social Development.

Krogh, K., J. Johnson and T. Bowman. (2003). *The Politics of Accountability: Home Support and Citizenship for People with Disabilities.* Unpublished manuscript, Ryerson University, School of Disability Studies.

Kvetoslava, R. (1999). *Personal Assistance – A Key Toward Independence in the Life of People with Severe Disabilities in Slovakia.* (Report of the Ministry of Labour, Social Affairs and Family of the Slovak Republic).

Lakey, J. (1994). *Caring About Independence: Disabled People and the Independent Living Fund.* London, UK: Policy Studies Institute.

Linton, S. (1998). *Claiming Disability: Knowledge and Identity.* New York: New York University Press.

Malhotra, Ravi. (2001). "Tracy Latimer, Disability Rights and the Left." *Canadian Dimension, 35,* 23-25.

Masuda, S. (1998). *The Impact of Block Funding on Women with Disabilities.* Ottawa, Ontario: DisAbled Women's Network Canada.

Meekosha, H. (1999). "Body Battles: Bodies, Gender and Disability," p.163-197 in T. Shakespeare (ed.), *The Disability Reader: Social Science Perspectives.* New York: Cassell.

Meekosha, H. and L. Dowse. (1997, Autumn). "Enabling Citizenship: Gender, Disability and Citizenship in Australia." *Feminist Review, 57,* 49-72.

Morgan, C. (1995). *Family Resources Survey Great Britain 1993/94.* London: Department of Social Security.

Morris, J. (1993). *Independent Lives? Community Care and Disabled People.* Basingstoke,UK: Macmillan.

——— (2001). "Impairment and Disability: Constructing an Ethic of Care that Promotes Human Rights." *Hypatia,* 16(4), 1-16.

Morris, M. (2001). *Community Care and Caregiving Research: A Synthesis Paper.* Ottawa: Women's Health Bureau, Health Canada and The Home and Continuing Care Unit, Health Care Directorate, Health Canada, and the Status of Women Canada.

National Alliance for Care Giving and the American Association of Retired Persons. (1997). *Family Care Giving in the U.S.: Findings From a National Survey* (Final Report). Bethesda, MD: National Alliance for Care Giving.

Oliver, M. (1992). "Changing the Social Relations of Research Production?" *Disability, Handicap and Society, 7,* 101-114.

——— (1996a). *Understanding Disability: From Theory to Practice.* Basingstoke, UK: Macmillan.

Orme, J. (2001). *Gender and Community Care: Social Work and Social Care Perspectives.* Basingstoke, UK: Palgrave.

O'Toole, C.J. and T. Doe. (2002). "Sexuality and Disabled Parents with Disabled Children." *Sexuality and Disability,* 30(1), 89-101.

Pirie, M. (1988). "Women and Illness Role: Rethinking Feminist Theory." *Canadian Review of Sociology and Anthropology, 25,* 628-648.

Pollak, N. and M. Cohen (eds.). (2000). *Without Foundation* (Report produced by Canadian Centre for Policy Alternatives–BC Office, British Columbia Government and Service Employees' Union, British Columbia Nurses' Union and Hospital Employees' Union). Vancouver, BC: Canadian Centre for Policy Alternatives.

Priestley, M. (1998). "Discourse and Resistance in Care Assessment: Integrated Living and Community Care." *British Journal of Social Work, 28,* 659-673.

——— (1999). *Disability Politics and Community Care.* Philadelphia: Jessica Kingsley.

Proctor, G. (2001). "Listening to Older Women with Dementia: Relationships, Voices and Power." *Disability and Society,* 16(3), 361-376.

Putnam, R.D. (1993, Spring). "The Prosperous Community: Social Capital and Public Life." *The American Prospect* 4(13). Retrieved 6 May 2003 from http://www.prospect.org/print/V4/13/putnam-r.html

Rachlis, M. and C. Kushner (1994). *Strong Medicine: How to Save Canada's Health Care System*. Toronto: Harper Collins.

Razack, S. (1999). *Looking White People in the Eye: Gender, Race and Culture in the Courtrooms and Classrooms*. Toronto, Ontario: University of Toronto Press.

Rioux, M.H. (1997). "Disability: The Place of Judgment in a World of Fact." *Journal of Intellectual Disability Research,* 41(part 2), 101-111.

Roeher Institute. (1995). *Disability Supports: Patterns in Usage and Need Among Adult Canadians with Disabilities* (Report). Toronto, Ontario.

Roeher Institute and Status of Women Canada. (2001, February). *Disability-related Support Arrangements, Policy Options, and Implications for Women's Equality* (Report prepared by the Roeher Institute for Status of Women Canada). Retrieved 6 May 2003, from the Status of Women Canada Web site: http://www.swc-cfc.gc.ca/pubs/0662653238/200102_0662653238_e.html

Saxton, M., M.A. Curry, L.E. Powers, S. Maley, K. Eckels and J. Gross. (2001). "Bring my Scooter so I Can Leave You: A Study of Disabled Women Handling Abuse by Personal Assistance Providers." *Violence Against Women,* 7, 393-417.

Schultz, R. and S.R. Beach. (1999). "Caregiving as a Risk Factor for Mortality: The Caregiver Health Effects Study." *Journal of the American Medical Association,* 282, 2215-2219.

Shakespeare, T. (2000). *Help.* Birmingham: Venture Press.

Snow, J. (1992). "Living at Home," p. 80-86 in D. Driedger and S. Gray (eds.), *Imprinting our Image: An International Anthology by Women with Disabilities*. Charlottetown, Prince Edward Island: Gynergy Books.

Sobsey, D. and T. Doe. (1991). "Patterns of Sexual Abuse and Assault." *Disability and Sexuality, 9,* 243-259.

Statistics Canada. (2001a). *Canadian Community Health Survey, 2000-2001*. Ottawa, Ontario: Health Statistics Division, Government of Canada.

———— (2001b). *Participation and Activity Limitation Survey, 2001: A Profile of Disability in Canada*. Ottawa, Ontario: Government of Canada.

Thomas, P.G. (1996). "Visions Versus Resources in the Federal Program Review," p. 39-46 in A. Armit and J. Bourgault (eds.), *Hard Choices or no Choices: Assessing Program Review*. Toronto, Ontario: Institute of Public Administration of Canada.

Tighe, C.A. (2001). "Working at Disability: A Qualitative Study of the Meaning of Health and Disability for Women with Physical Impairments." *Disability and Society,* 16, 511-529.

Trypuc, J.M. (1994). "Gender Based Mortality and Morbidity Patterns and Health Risks," in B. Singh Bolaria and R. Bolaria (eds.), *Women, Medicine, and Health*. Halifax, Nova Scotia: Fernwood.

Tuohy, C.J. (1992). *Policy and Politics in Canada: Institutionalized Ambivalence*. Philadelphia: Temple University Press.

Twig, J. (2000). *Bathing: The Body and Community Care*. London: Routledge.

Walmsley, J. (1993) "Talking to Top People: Some Issues Related to the Citizenship of People with Learning Disabilities," p. 257-266 in J. Swain, V. Finkelstein, S. French and M. Oliver (eds.), *Disabling Barriers: Enabling Environments*. London, UK: Sage in association with Open University.

Wendell, S. (1996). *The Rejected Body: Feminist Philosophical Reflections on Disability*. New York: Routledge.

Wendell, S. (2001). "Unhealthy Disabled: Treating Chronic Illnesses as Disabilities." *Hypatia,* 16(4), 17-33.

Williamson, G.M., D.R. Shaffer and R. Schultz. (1998). "Activity Restriction and Prior Relationship History as Contributors to Mental Health Outcomes Among Middle-aged and Older Spouse Caregivers." *Health Psychology,* 17, 152-162.

World Health Organization. (2001). *International Classification of Functioning, Disability and Health (ICF)*. Retrieved 6 May 2003, from the World Health Organization Web site: http://www3.who.int/icf/icftemplate.cfm

Wuest, J. (1993). "Institutionalizing Women's Oppression: The Inherent Risk in Health Policy that Fosters Community Participation." *Health Care for Women International,* 14, 407-417.

Young, I.M. (1990). *Justice and the Politics of Difference.* Princeton, NJ: Princeton University Press.

———— (2000). "Disability and the Definition of Work." p. 169-173 in L. Francis and A. Silvers (eds.), *Americans with Disabilities: Exploring Implications of the Law for Individuals and Institutions.* New York: Routledge.

Yuval-Davis, N. (1997). "Women, Citizenship and Difference." *Feminist Review,* 57, 4-27.

Aboriginal Women and Home Care

Shelley Thomas Prokop, Erika Haug, Michelle Hogan,
Jason McCarthy, and Lorraine MacDonald

INTRODUCTION

Aboriginal women have always played a central role as caregivers and healers within their families and communities. Over the course of their lives, many Aboriginal women will go back and forth between being care providers and requiring care themselves. As is the case with other Canadian women, providing care has been a taken-for-granted part of Aboriginal women's unpaid work in the home. While women in Canada provide 80 percent of caregiving, which includes both paid and unpaid work, the gender discrepancy is arguably even higher in Aboriginal communities, due to a number of factors including cultural values of caring for family members, lack of services and lack of professional training opportunities.

The availability of home care services is particularly important to Aboriginal women for many reasons. First, many Aboriginal women with disabilities, activity limitations and chronic health problems could benefit from home care services that would enable them to remain at home and participate in their communities. Second, as care providers, women are affected – often adversely – by the care needs of others and their access to appropriate health services. Third, home care is important to Aboriginal women because alternatives to home care, such as institutional care, may not exist in their communities or may not be acceptable due to lack of cultural congruence.

Aboriginal people have repeatedly identified the importance of providing home care services that enable them to remain in their own communities where they can continue their culture and traditions. More than a decade ago, a report prepared by the Federation of Saskatchewan Indian Nations (FSIN) entitled *Homecare on Reserve: A Framework,* included this Elders' vision of home care: "The vision of the Elders, handicapped and chronically and acutely ill, is to continue to live productive, useful lives in their homes, close to their families, in their communities … and (to) help maintain culture, language and traditions … Their vision for home-care on-reserve is a guarantee that (First) Nations will have the authority and finances to help them live and contribute always to their communities" (1990:7).

While home care providers and recipients have already been identified as marginalized by the policy-making process (Morris 2001) Aboriginal women are one of the most politically, socially and economically marginalized populations in Canada. They experience multiple barriers to participating in broader policy decisions that directly affect their lives. Aboriginal women experience chronic diseases, poverty and systemic discrimination at a much higher level than the general Canadian population. At the same time, they bring unique knowledge and expertise, based on traditional holistic understandings of health, to the domain of home care. Therefore, it is extremely important that Aboriginal women become not just objects but subjects of home care policy and program development, so that home care programming can be shaped by their culture, values, aspirations, healing gifts, vision and understandings of health.

To date, the literature on home care in Canada has failed to include any studies focused specifically on Aboriginal women's experiences as home care providers and recipients. No studies explore their unique experiences as formal (paid) home care providers, informal (unpaid) caregivers or care recipients. Also, there remains a major gap in terms of policies and programs which specifically address home care training, employment and service provision for Aboriginal women. It has been recognized that caregivers and care recipients in Aboriginal and other minority communities face racism, language and cultural barriers that make them more disadvantaged and less well served than others (Morris 2002). However, there has been no further investigation into how these barriers affect Aboriginal women's experiences of home care. Aboriginal women are largely absent from the research on gender and home care, and home care is largely absent from the research on Aboriginal women's health.

Given this lack of research and literature, this chapter will provide a context for exploring Aboriginal women's relationship to home care, in the hope of raising questions that can be explored in future research. The chapter provides a profile of Aboriginal women's health that has implications for Aboriginal women's needs for home care services. In addition, the recent development of the First Nations and Inuit Home and Community Care Program, and the training and employment opportunities for women associated with this program, are discussed. From this discussion, we will reflect on some of the current challenges and opportunities in the area of Aboriginal home care delivery. Finally, we will recommend policy, program, research and education strategies that can be employed to address the current challenges identified.

Towards a Working Definition of
Aboriginal Home Care

Before we can address the question of "What is Aboriginal home care?" we must first clarify the language used for this discussion. According to the *Canadian Oxford Dictionary* (2001) the term Aboriginal refers to all people "inhabiting or existing in a land from the earliest times or from before the arrival of colonists." In practice, through colonial policies, Aboriginal people have been subdivided into the categories Indian, Inuit and Métis. Indian people are further subdivided as either status or non-status, and status people are designated as either treaty or non-treaty. The term First Nations is politically, historically and culturally more appropriate than the terms Native or Indian, but is not inclusive of all Aboriginal peoples as it excludes all non-status Aboriginal people. In this chapter we will generally speak of *Aboriginal* home care (rather than First Nations home care) to include all Indian, Inuit and Métis people.

Home care has been described as comprising two streams: "Professional services, such as nursing, occupational therapy and physiotherapy; and home support services, such as homemaking, personal care, housekeeping, and transportation. In addition, home care may include adult day programs, meal programs, home maintenance, respite care, medical equipment and supplies, and counseling" (Browne 2000:81). Both streams are relevant to Aboriginal home care, which seeks to define this broad spectrum of services in a culturally congruent manner.

For our purposes we will use the following working definition: "Aboriginal home care is formal health care services provided to members of Aboriginal communities in the space of their homes, in a culturally congruent manner." Aboriginal home care should not necessarily be provided solely by Aboriginal people. Rather, it is recognized that people who share belief systems, culture, traditions, language and a way of life bring a level of comfort and understanding that is immeasurable to Aboriginal home care recipients, allowing care to take place in a calm, soothing and supportive environment.

> Aboriginal home care must be considered holistically to encompass an array of services enabling people to live at home, with the effect of promoting health, preventing disease, encouraging support and rehabilitative care, and preventing, delaying, or substituting long term or acute care alternatives. Home care which maximizes overall health and one's own sense of well being; care that facilitates participation in community life; care that is consistent with the notions of social citizenship and the basic right of dignity; and care that is directed by those receiving it. (Butot et al. 2002:12)

If we define Aboriginal home care as formal health care services, we must then consider what is meant by *health care*, and *health*. According to Aboriginal world views, health is understood as a holistic balance between the physical, spiritual, mental and emotional aspects of a person. The circle is used to represent the inseparability of the individual from their family, community and the world. It also represents harmony and balance in all aspects of a person's physical and social environment. Balance is considered essential to live, grow and reach one's full potential as a human being. This interconnectedness is an integral philosophical concept that was common to the many different Aboriginal peoples who lived throughout North America (Abele 1989:205).

The model of the medicine wheel, used primarily by the Cree people, provides a physical representation of First Nations philosophy. This model also represents a key framework for exploring Aboriginal understanding of health, in terms of both diagnosis and treatment. The medicine wheel is an ancient symbol of the universe used to help people understand ideas that cannot be seen physically. It reflects the cosmic order, the unity of all things and represents the circle of life in all its forms and manifestations. It is a tool for teaching, an instrument of understanding and it manifests itself into a way of thinking. It is life itself (Grey Wolf 2000:24).

According to Aboriginal world views, healing cannot occur in the physical body without addressing and bringing into alignment the other aspects of one's being. Nor can an individual's healing occur in isolation from the rest of the community: human, spiritual and ecological. An individual's healing requires not just medical treatment but also the spiritual support and strength of family, community and cultural traditions. Rather than healing being an occasional physical transformation, for Aboriginal people it is a way of life. Illness is understood as falling out of balance and losing the connection to the Creator's instructions for living the good life, so various ceremonies are used by traditional healers to realign the lives of individuals who seek healing. Two such ceremonies are the sweatlodge and fasting, both of which are designed to reconnect individuals with the Creator.

Caregiving for family members has always been an integral aspect of Aboriginal philosophy and, because these values and structures are strong, many Aboriginal people have needed very little outside assistance in caring for those who are sick or in need of long-term care. Aboriginal communities also have rich traditions of healing and knowledge of health that inform their caregiving. In their book *Medicine Women, Curanderas, and Women Doctors*, Perrone et al. note that: "the history of contributions by Native American cultures (hundreds of them) to modern healing techniques and knowledge has not been widely known" (1989:21). At the time of contact, Aboriginal people on this continent "knew more about anatomy and the treatment of trauma and illness than the average European, and in some respects, more than European physicians" (1989:22). Aboriginal women have frequently been the carriers of this traditional knowledge and have played prominent roles as community healers throughout the generations.

In 1980 the federal government proclaimed on a national and international level the importance of incorporating traditional healing practices into the health care services provided to Aboriginal people, yet concrete follow-through on this intent has been lacking (Gregory 1988:42). Aboriginal home care is a potential space where traditional Aboriginal knowledge systems and paradigms of health could be combined with the Euro-Canadian bio-medical model which currently underlies health care and home care delivery. This fusion of health care paradigms can occur in a *syncretic* fashion, as "a fusion or union of originally differing and even conflicting components" (Perrone et al. 1989:4).

HISTORICAL AND ENVIRONMENTAL CONTEXT
OF ABORIGINAL HOME CARE

According to Aboriginal world views, neither individuals nor programs can be looked at apart from their ecological, social, spiritual and physical environments. Nor can they be separated from their historical context. We therefore cannot fully understand Aboriginal women's experiences with home care without examining the broader environmental and historical context in which their experiences are embedded.

The challenges currently faced by Aboriginal women and their communities are inextricably linked to five centuries of colonization, assimilation and marginalization. European contact brought diseases previously unknown to the inhabitants of Turtle Island – huge numbers of indigenous people lost their lives in epidemics of diseases to which they had no immunity. This initial devastation was followed by the European quest for land. Aboriginal people were seen as obstacles to progress and settlement and so the state developed a tripartite policy of protection, civilization and assimilation (Milloy 1978). Government-funded and church-delivered residential schools played a key role in carrying out this agenda by removing generations of children from their languages, cultures and families.

Aboriginal women's traditional position of respect and honour was greatly damaged by the imposition of patriarchy through Christianity, the shift to a market-based economy and colonial legislation such as *The Indian Act* which undermined Aboriginal women's economic, political and social roles in their communities. Residential schools, in particular, were a powerful socialization force in training women to be passive, submissive and voiceless.

The long-term effects of residential schools, coupled with generations of grief and feelings of dispossession dating back to contact, manifest themselves through the generations in various ways: dehumanization and alienation, cultural schizophrenia, low self-esteem and confidence, self-hate and feelings of inferiority, apathy and lethargy, and feelings of hopelessness. These symptoms, combined with paternalistic state policies that have disempowered Aboriginal communities and disassembled traditional health systems and structures based on ceremonies outlawed in the *Indian Act*, contribute directly to increases in physical, mental and spiritual health problems.

Many Aboriginal people have felt that the Euro-Canadian model of health care, as guided by the *Canada Health Act*, which ensures provision only for acute care services offered by medical doctors and hospital systems, is incongruent and sometimes incompatible with Aboriginal understandings of health and illness. Many Aboriginal women report being poorly served by the bio-medical approach to health care (Perrone et al. 1989). Browne et al. (2000) advocated policies to protect Aboriginal women from the institutional discrimination in contemporary health care systems. Otherwise, they would be left with little reason to fully trust the services.

Others argue that the high rate of disease in Aboriginal communities reflects the inability of the bio-medical health care system to effectively meet the needs of Aboriginal people. This sense of dispossession from the mainstream health system is also reflected in lower levels of Aboriginal people's participation within the health care system. Currently only 6.2 percent of Aboriginal women in the workforce are part of the health sector, as compared to 8.7 percent for non-Aboriginals. In Inuit and reserve communities these rates are even lower, with the Inuit rate being 3.4 percent and the reserve population rate being 3.7 percent (Statistics Canada 2002). If this situation is to change, "[H]ealth reform must also focus on policies that address those critical determinants of health, including: the absence of discrimination, social justice to prevent systemic discrimination and health inequalities, and social relationships that respect diversity. Examining the ways in which these determinants can be addressed through policy will require meaningful involvement of Aboriginal women who are affected by such policies" (Browne et al. 2000:29).

Health Status of Aboriginal Women
Life expectancy for Aboriginal women in Canada is 76 years, or five years less than that of non-Aboriginal women (Health Canada 2002). This shorter life expectancy is a reflection of the persistent inequalities in health status and the higher rates of illness and injury among the Aboriginal population as a whole. Poorer health, higher rates of chronic diseases, higher rates of disabilities and an increase in the aging population all contribute to the need for home care services in Aboriginal communities.

Aboriginal women experience many conditions that would be improved by health education, assistance with activities of daily living, home support services and home nursing care, as well as traditional healing practices. They have higher rates of circulatory problems, respiratory diseases, diabetes, hypertension and cancer of the cervix than non-Aboriginal women do (Health Canada 2002). Similarly, the self-reported incidence of chronic diseases among First Nations and Inuit women is higher than in the non-Aboriginal population: 2.5 times higher for heart problems and hypertension, 1.5 times higher for arthritis and rheumatism, 1.6 times higher for cancer and 5.3 times higher for diabetes (Health Canada 1999a:7). Many of those with chronic diseases report activity limitations (24).

Rates of diabetes among Aboriginal women are increasing at an alarming pace. Diabetes affects one in three Aboriginal women over the age of 55 (Reading 1999:48). We know that type 2 diabetes is connected to obesity and that 60 percent of adult Aboriginal women are considered obese (Health Canada 1999:20). If the incidence rate remains unchanged, the number of diabetic Aboriginals in Manitoba, for example, will be 27 percent by 2016. (Encouragingly, the rate of juvenile or insulin dependent diabetes [type 1] for Aboriginals is approximately the same as that of the non-Aboriginal population.)

Aboriginal women, on average, experience disabilities at twice the rate of non-Aboriginal women. For children and young adults, the rate is three times higher (AFN 2000:1). Since women are the primary caregivers for children and other family members with disabilities, lack of access to adequate services for persons with disabilities can have a directly negative affect on women as caregivers, as well as direct recipients of care.

First Nations and Inuit elders experienced more heart problems, high blood pressure, diabetes, arthritis and rheumatism than other Canadians of the same age (Health Canada 1999a:7). One in four are limited in their activities in the home and one in eight is unable to leave the home and requires home care. According to the National Advisory Council on Aging, older Aboriginal people experience disability for over twice as long as do non-Aboriginal people (Health Canada 1999:24). While elders currently comprise only 4 percent of the Aboriginal population, it is anticipated that this rate will increase to 7 percent by 2016 (Health Canada 2000a). Buchignani and Armstrong-Esther note that "extensive dependence on informal care, institutional barriers and local service unavailability lead Native seniors to under-utilize other formal programs aimed generically at the older provincial population" (1999:3) thus further underlining the importance of Aboriginal home care.

Economic and Physical Environment: Poverty

Poverty represents one of the greatest negative impacts on Aboriginal women's well-being. Its multiple impacts include limited access to transportation, low self-esteem, poor diet, stress due to inadequate and crowded housing, and limited resources to provide for families. Aboriginal women are more likely to get sick and to stay sicker longer living in conditions of poverty.

The average income for Aboriginal people aged 15-65 years old is $17,823, or one-third less than the general population which averages $25,435. The extent of poverty among Aboriginal women is particularly severe. Satzewich and Wotherspoon (2000:103) note that one-quarter of Aboriginal women have no income, compared with 13 percent of Aboriginal men, 19 percent of all Canadian women and 7 percent of all Canadian men.

Housing inequities and substandard housing also have a direct impact on Aboriginal women's lives as caregivers and care-receivers and represent a particular barrier for those with physical limitations. Inadequate housing for Aboriginal peoples is just one manifestation of the policy failure of the federal and provincial/territorial governments. Although the federal government reports that the number of houses on-reserve increased by 13 percent between 1996 and 2000 (INAC 2003) the AFN stresses that the housing situation on reserves remains critical in terms of overcrowding, poor construction and inadequate numbers of houses. For example, the AFN states that more than 28 percent of housing on-reserve requires major repairs. Furthermore, the rate of tuberculosis in First Nations and Inuit communities, although in decline, is still 18 times that of the general population and has been directly connected to the overcrowded housing conditions in First Nations communities (Health Canada 1999:7).

Ecological Environment: Environmental Racism

In addition to living with the challenges of substandard housing in their immediate physical environments, Aboriginal women face disproportionate health risks from their ecological environment. Environmental health refers to how our health is affected by contaminants in our environment (e.g., air pollution, toxic chemicals, waste disposal). Contaminants include dioxins and furans, PCBs, metals and DDT. Harmful effects from contaminants include cancer, contamination of breast milk, birth defects, child developmental problems, stomach illness and respiratory illness (Health Canada 1999b). Environmental racism refers to the disproportionate concentration of environmental toxins around indigenous, and culturally and economically marginalized, populations with little political influence.

When environmental contaminants build up in the body tissues of fish and game, they become concentrated in human tissue. Because indigenous peoples in Canada consume fish and wild meat at a higher rate than the general population does, environmental toxins have disproportionately affected their health. For example, PCBs and mercury are significant health hazards in First Nation and Inuit communities, particularly for child development and the immune system. On Broughton Island, Nunavut, 60 percent of children and 40 percent of women of childbearing age have PCB burdens exceeding tolerable limits (Health Canada 1999b:18). Quebec Inuit and Montagnais newborns have PCB burdens "over the threshold beyond which cognitive impairments were expected to result" (18). There is evidence that women who eat large amounts of Great Lakes fish have children who are smaller than average and are physically and mentally delayed (Health Canada 1999b). The James Bay Cree were found to have mercury levels as high as 15.0 mg/kg when health risks are associated with levels of only 1mg/kg (18). These statistics are only a sample of the environmental health risks faced by (particularly northern) Aboriginal people. This discussion may have an impact on home care service provision because, if people are living in toxic environments that are making them sick, home care – even if it is culturally appropriate and accessible – will only ever be a superficial band-aid.

Spiritual and Political Environment:
Retrenchment of Both Health Care and Treaty
Rights and Cultural Revival

Through the treaty-making process that occurred in the 1800s, the Crown agreed to provide First Nations with health care, housing and education in exchange for the vast tracks of ceded land. Today, reserve land makes up less than 5 percent of Canada's total land mass. Many people on reserves are living in Third World conditions in terms of health, housing and poverty. Where First Nations people envisioned comprehensive health care provisions, the federal government has focused on controlling and reducing the levels of health care expenditures through devolution, downloading and restricting access to services (Frideres 1998). As Siemens notes,

> The government continues to deny its fiduciary responsibilities to provide comprehensive health services (to Aboriginal people). Rather, we see an erosion of health services under the auspices of what the government calls a move to self-determination. The government claims to be giving responsibility and support back to the Aboriginal community. However, they are expected to do more with less, as exemplified by the shifting of responsibility from the federal level to the Aboriginal community level. (2003: 11-12)

Today, as part of a larger cultural and linguistic revival occurring across Canada, a cultural renaissance is occurring in the area of health care, whereby Aboriginal people are seeking to *indigenize* service systems (Waldram 1995). This renaissance is occurring in relation to concomitant trends of retrenchment of both the health care system and treaty rights for Aboriginal people. The politics of home care can thus be seen to represent only a small piece of the broader challenge for Aboriginal people to gain self-determination of health care programming. As Elias et al. note, "Health promotion is also very much about self-governance. Although non-governmental bodies are eager to act on behalf of First Nations in the field of health promotion by creating opportunities to advance First Nation voices, such actions can still be interpreted as another form of cultural imperialism. Promoting First Nation health from a holistic view is an act of First Nation self-governance, which requires a First Nation perspective" (2000:5).

Despite the tremendous challenges, Aboriginal women today are claiming their voice and positions as leaders and healers within their communities. They are becoming increasingly politically active, particularly within their own government structures, and are pushing for social and gender issues that are often marginalized by male-dominated leadership. As Browne et al. state, "when we view the tensions between the First Nations and the dominant sites of power as structural communication, it is evident that the power imbalances that give rise to the women's concerns regarding their health care cannot be redressed without radical changes in the political relations" (2000:27).

Many examples of Aboriginal women taking leadership in the domain of health care can be found across the country. For example, the Federation of Saskatchewan Indians has a Saskatchewan First Nations Women's Council (SFNWC) consisting of elected Women Chiefs and The Women's Leadership, which is made up of approximately 95 elected women Councillors. These women are committed to addressing issues that affect women in Aboriginal communities, including home care. On a national level, the Native Women's Association of Canada (NWAC) was formed "to help empower women by being involved in developing and changing legislation which affects them, and by involving them in the development and delivery of programs promoting equal opportunity for Aboriginal women" (NWAC Web site). As well, in 1998 the Office of the Senior Advisor on Aboriginal Women's Issues and Gender Equality was established by Indian Affairs and Northern Development Canada and is assisted by a department-wide Advisory Committee on Gender Equality, including representatives from both regional offices and headquarters (Status of Women Canada 2001:19).

A REVIEW OF ABORIGINAL HOME CARE DELIVERY PROGRAMS

The Assembly of First Nations (AFN) has been lobbying since 1988 for First Nations home care programs. In 1998, their efforts were rewarded by an 18-month pilot project called the *"Home and Community Care Program."* The goal of the program was to provide basic home and community care services that are comprehensive, effective and accessible to Aboriginal people. "The program was described as an approach aimed at transferring power and jurisdiction to Aboriginal people based upon the concept of self-determination ... It was felt that changes needed to occur at the community level" (Siemens 2003:3). The services were to be culturally sensitive and responsive to the unique needs of First Nations and Inuit communities while being comparable in quality to similar services provided to other Canadians. The project was supported by Health Canada, received its primary funding from the Health Transition Fund and was administered by the newly created First Nations and Inuit Home and Community Care Program.

Following the initial pilot project, the AFN lobbied the federal government to increase its commitment to First Nations home care. On 23 July 1999, the AFN issued a First Nations Home Care Resolution that emphasized the federal government's fiduciary responsibility to provide home care as an element of health care rights. The resolution stated:

> *"Whereas* there is a growing need in First Nation communities for Home and Continuing Care/Special Care services because of high rates of chronic illness, aging of the population, high rates of disabilities and the impact of provincial health reforms," and

> *"Whereas* First Nations must have adequate resources to ensure Elders/ special needs persons can remain in their communities as they age so that their knowledge and wisdom can be shared with the youth, and that they can be treated with the proper respect."

> *"Be it resolved that*: Immediate new federal resources be made available to meet the current crisis in First Nations Home Care/ Special Care, and that this be recognized on a need basis as opposed to the current population funding formula from [Medical Services Branch]/ INAC ... [and] The rights of Elders/elders/special needs persons to plan, design, deliver and control services must be respected."

Thus, from the initial pilot project and resolutions put forth by the AFN, a framework for Aboriginal home care design and delivery was established. A "First Nations and Inuit Home and Community Care Planning Resource Kit" was compiled to outline clearly the process for planning and implementing home care in other First Nations and Inuit communities. Today, any First Nation or Inuit community with a population of more than 500 and which is affiliated with a tribal council or Inuit Association, can apply for funding to create their own home care program. Funding through the First Nations and Inuit Home and Community Care Program is available for core planning, service delivery, health training and capital construction and equipment.

The services provided by the First Nations and Inuit Home and Community Care Program include client assessment, case management, home care nursing, personal care, and home support. Certified aides supervised by a nurse provide these latter home care services. Some communities also provide other services, including in-home respite, palliative care, client advocacy, Elders' activity centres, foot care for clients with diabetes, monthly shopping programs, therapeutic bath programs, adult day programs, meal programs, lifelines, woodcutting, water hauling, Elders' community dinners and Elders' activity gatherings (Health Canada 2000:55-74). This program also offers home-based services for clients with psychiatric, mental or emotional health problems. Some of these services may include traditional healing (Health Canada 2001b). Since the framework for Aboriginal home care is structured to allow optimal community control, it is not monolithic, rather, it takes different forms depending on which community is developing the programs and services. As a result, a wide range of creative home care programming has developed across Canada in response to the unique needs of various communities.

The inclusion of traditional healing, Elders' community dinners, water hauling, and woodcutting in home care programs demonstrates the attempt to design programs that are culturally appropriate and responsive to community needs. Nevertheless, in the preliminary evaluations of these pilot projects, there is no particular mention of the fact that Aboriginal women and men may have different home care needs or may be affected differently by the provision of home care services.

Another result of the initial Aboriginal home care project was an 18-month home care program designed specifically to respond to the increasing prevalence of diabetes in four Aboriginal communities. The project's goals were to identify ways to expand diabetes care and treatment support through home and community care services, and to share these models for service delivery with other communities. The results demonstrated an effective and positive approach to community-based diabetes care (Health Canada 1999).

GAPS IN ABORIGINAL HOME CARE PROGRAMS

Regardless of where a person lives, whether she speaks an Aboriginal language or not, or how much her Aboriginal ancestry is apparent, the single greatest determinant of an Aboriginal person's access to health, social, or educational services, including Aboriginal home care, is how this person has been categorized by the federal government. As a result of these classifications, Aboriginal women living in the same or nearby communities may have completely different access to services. Although the multiple classifications developed in the 1800s are confusing and archaic, divisive and demeaning, they continue today because the federal government is reluctant to acknowledge its financial responsibilities towards all Aboriginal people.

For Inuit and First Nations (status) people, the First Nations Inuit Health Branch (FNIHB) of the federal government still holds responsibility for the provision of all health care services including home care. Due to the historical policy of keeping First Nations people on their reserves, the federal government focuses the bulk of its health programming on reserves. Off-reserve First Nations and Métis people generally fall under provincial jurisdiction for home care services, while on-reserve, non-status persons are in danger of falling through the cracks in terms of service coverage.

The restricted coverage of federal Aboriginal health programs is evident in the First Nations and Inuit Home and Community Care Program. This program is only available to status populations living on-reserve, in Inuit settlements, or in communities north of the 60th parallel. The First Nations and Inuit Home and Community Care Program excludes the Métis population and 53 percent of the First Nations population that lives off-reserve, even though they may have similar needs for culturally appropriate services. Of First Nations people, 24 percent live in urban areas, 29 percent live in rural areas and 47 percent live on-reserve (Statistics Canada 2003:12).

First Nations women have been drawn to urban centres by the convergence of several factors, including greater participation in post-secondary education, lack of economic opportunities on reserves, and domestic abuse and violence (INAC 2002:8). For Aboriginal people living off-reserve, the federal government has stated that they should receive home care services from provincial health services or municipal services such as health regions or districts (Siemens 2003:13). The current trend towards privatization of home care services, which is leading to increases in user fees, uneven standards of service delivery and lower salaries for home care providers (Browne 2000) disproportionately harms Aboriginal women who are not status and/or located on reserves.

A recent report released by the First Nations and Inuit Regional Health Survey National Steering Committee noted that current alternatives to institutional care, like home care, "are not offered or are inaccessible to the vast majority of First Nations and the Inuit. In addition, existing funding levels are inadequate and generate further inequalities and much criticism" (Reading 1999:149). Furthermore, the report noted that: "the cohort requiring home care services is increasing, and First Nations do not have the same access as other Canadians to re-investments in more complex and comprehensive home care services. Current programs and resources available to First Nations and Inuit cannot absorb the increased demands for home care services" (First Nations and Inuit Health Branch 2003:16).

TRAINING ABORIGINAL WOMEN IN HOME CARE:
ISSUES AND CHALLENGES

Several home care training programs have been designed since 1988 to meet the specific needs of Aboriginal students, the vast majority of whom are women. These training programs have required creative adaptations in terms of curriculum design, entrance requirements and modes of delivery. They have been largely welcomed as a positive development, resulting in increased training and employment opportunities for women, financial compensation for care work previously done without pay, and increased quality of care. However, the shift has not been without tensions, complexities and challenges, including: formal education levels of students, English as a Second Language (ESL) language barriers, accessibility, high cost of providing training and the question of how indigenization of home care actually happens. These challenges have been particularly pronounced for residents of rural and remote communities.

A common challenge for these programs to resolve has been lower formal education levels of potential students in respect of educational requirements based on Euro-Canadian contexts and standards. While many potential students bring a wealth of life experience and expertise as caregivers and healers in their communities, their formal education levels are often significantly lower than the general Canadian population because of multiple interlinking factors of colonization, including inferior formal education from residential schools and poverty. About 14 percent of Aboriginal women hold a university degree, while 30 percent have training in the trades, 38 percent have a grade 9-13 level of education and 17 percent have less than a grade nine education. In comparison, about 21 percent of non-Aboriginal women hold a university degree, while 28 percent have training in the trades, 46 percent have a grade 9-13 level of education and 14 percent have less than a grade nine education. Among the Inuit, only 5 percent of women hold a university degree, while 13 percent of Métis women and 12 percent of reserve Aboriginal people are university graduates (Statistics Canada 2002) (all figures rounded off). Aboriginal home care programs must consider how to address these realities.

The minimum entrance requirement for most home care programs is grade 12, which poses a major barrier to the 17 percent of Aboriginal women who hold less than a grade nine education and who are also the most likely to stay long-term in their communities. Consequently, several home care programs designed specifically for Aboriginal students have adapted their entrance requirements. One example is the Yukon College, which offers a 24-week *Home Support Worker/Nursing Home Attendant* program. And Aurora College in the Northwest Territories offers a *Home and Community Support Worker* program that integrates traditional Aboriginal knowledge. The Aurora program is directed at students 18 years of age or older with a minimal education of grade ten, or who are able to read and write English at a grade eight level, and/or who are mature students with relevant work experience. The course is broken down into three modules along with three practicum placements, and is offered through distance education training to meet the needs of the smaller communities in the Northwest Territories.

Other innovative programs have sprung up across Western Canada. The Saskatchewan Indian Institute of Technology (SIIT) was the first site in Canada to offer a Home Health Aide Program specifically for Aboriginal students. The SIIT program is designed to provide students with the essential learning experiences required to function efficiently and competently as health service workers in First Nation communities. Similarly, Camosun College in B.C. provides a First Nations Family Support Worker Program. The graduates of this program are qualified to work as part of a health team in Aboriginal communities under supervision by other professionals. The course is 10 months in length and provides credits that can be transferred to the Home Support/ Residential Care Attendant Program of the College. Kwantlen University College in B.C. also offers a Caregiver Educational Series program for those who provide caregiving to their family members. The curriculum takes a strong community-based approach, with an emphasis on addressing the sense of isolation and lack of power many caregivers feel. These programs have consistently found that a community-based approach that incorporates training in the community is the most successful.

Language issues, particularly for those who live in remote and isolated communities, have also challenged the home care programs. The ability to communicate with health care providers in one's own language has been identified as particularly important to Aboriginal women who speak an Aboriginal language. While approximately 32 percent of Aboriginal people in Canada speak a mother tongue, 60 percent of those over the age of 75 use an Aboriginal language (Statistics Canada 2003). Fully two-thirds of the Inuit population speak Inuktitut as a mother tongue (Statistics Canada 2003). In 2000, of the estimated 227,285 persons living on reserves, 17.2 percent were located within areas that Indian and Northern Affairs Canada (INAC) refers to as special access zones. These zones are defined as communities "where a First Nation has no year-round road access to the nearest service centre and, as a result, experiences a higher cost of transportation" (INAC 2002:80). A further 3.7 percent live in a remote zone, which is defined as a community "where a First Nation is located over 350 km from the nearest service centre having year-round road access" (80). In special access and remote zones, a much higher percentage of the population speak Aboriginal languages and many older Aboriginal persons are not comfortable speaking English or French. Thus, if home care training programs are to be truly accessible, they must find ways to meet the needs of ESL and rural and remote Aboriginal students.

While all of these programs seek to provide training that is culturally congruent, there are different interpretations about what this actually means. In some contexts, it may simply mean changing the textbook examples from Euro-Canadian ones to Aboriginal ones. In this model Aboriginal people are delivering programs and services that are essentially based on non-Aboriginal models and world views. Others feel that a truly *indigenized* home care program must be clearly founded on Aboriginal world views, knowledge, beliefs and understandings of health and illness. This question will continue to underpin Aboriginal home care development and will be answered differently according to the different contexts in which training programs are developed.

While there are undoubtedly numerous benefits to the professionalization of home care services, the shift from informal to formal care provision cannot be naively assumed to be a unilateral good and critical questions must certainly be asked about its impact. Aboriginal home care can be seen as situated within a contested territory of power dynamics between different ways of knowing, between Western medical models and traditional indigenous concepts of health. What happens when there is a conflict between these two paradigms? Whose knowledge is represented and privileged in home care educational programs, and to what degree?

The professionalization of care can represent a shift away from traditional Aboriginal to bio-medical knowledge systems and market-based systems and structures. When services and systems embedded within an Aboriginal cultural context are transformed according to Euro-Canadian models of health care delivery, what is the impact on traditional healers, medicine people and midwives who have experienced centuries of colonial domination by Western medical, religious and social institutions (O'Neil 1988:29)? Furthermore, to what extent does home care training actually reinscribe gender oppression, taking Aboriginal women up one step from unpaid to paid caregiving, but keeping them restricted in an occupation that offers low salaries and little upward mobility or professional development opportunities (Browne 2000)?

RECOMMENDATIONS

As noted earlier in this chapter, there has been no literature produced on Aboriginal women and home care. As such, in light of our research, we have identified a number of recommendations that should be taken into consideration when addressing the training, programming, policy and research issues surrounding Aboriginal home care delivery, particularly by and for Aboriginal women.

Training

1. In view of the increasing needs for Aboriginal home care as discussed in this chapter, more culturally appropriate educational programs which provide in-depth training on how to effectively provide home care to Aboriginal people must be developed through consultation with Elders, who are the keepers of Aboriginal traditions.
2. It is important for the federal government to strengthen its educational funds to support Aboriginal women's integration into the health care sector, particularly for residents of remote and northern communities who face much greater expenses in accessing training. Support for female students within communities maximizes success in educational programs.

Programming

1. Aboriginal home care should be available as an inherent right rather than a special privilege, to *all* Aboriginal people, regardless of whether they have official status or live on-reserve or not. Therefore, jurisdictional problems related to home care service delivery must be resolved between Aboriginal leaders and representatives of various levels of government so that this right can be fully realized.
2. Further development of both on-and off-reserve Aboriginal home care services is urgently required to meet the present health needs of the Aboriginal population. Such development must actively incorporate the input of Elders and all community members affected by home care services. These home care services need to be culturally congruent, accessible and effective.
3. Federal, provincial/territorial and regional health authorities must recognize the long-term costs associated with the existing limited home care programs for Aboriginal people and increase their financial commitment to supporting capacity development of Aboriginal home care in urban and rural Aboriginal communities.
4. Aboriginal people in remote and special access areas must be given special consideration in view of the particular challenges they face in accessing formal home care services and training. Capacity building for home care development among remote populations will be particularly necessary to alleviate the multiple expenses incurred under the current system of service provision.

Policy

1. Gender considerations remain marginal to policy and program decision-making for Aboriginal home care. Policy changes need to be aimed at valuing the caregiving role and the experiences of women as recipients and providers of care.
2. As long as Aboriginal people continue to live in Third World conditions, there can be no effective home care. Therefore, in order for Aboriginal home care to be optimally effective, it is essential that outstanding land claims be resolved, that there be provision of adequate funds to Aboriginal communities for housing, health care, education and social development, and that environmental pollution of Aboriginal lands ceases so that traditional health systems can be maintained.
3. There is a direct need for coordination and communication between federal, provincial and territorial governments in regard to the programming needs of Aboriginal people. For example, the responsibility to meet the needs of First Nations and Inuit people being released from the hospital is a provincial/territorial matter. However, their aftercare is a federal matter. These services need to be better coordinated to ease the transition between hospital a stay and community integration.

4. In response to the Royal Commission on the Future of Health Care in Canada, it was proposed that a new piece of legislation, titled the *Canadian Continuum of Care Act*, be adopted, which would recognize non-hospital care and community support as integral to the health care system in Canada (Butot et al. 2002:10). Under this new act, care would follow the patient in either the home, the community or facility settings, whether acute or long term, and would ensure that all home care services are universally accessible and fully funded. Such legislation would directly benefit all Aboriginals, as well as all Canadians, in terms of increasing access to quality home care programming. It would also effectively address the threat posed by the privatization of home care services in terms of increasing user fees, uneven standards of service delivery and lower salaries for home care providers, all of which negatively impact Aboriginal women.

Research

1. The diverse and creative innovations occurring in the area of Aboriginal home care provision, and the impact of these programs on Aboriginal women as both recipients and providers of care, have yet to be studied and documented. Research projects that are action oriented, culturally sensitive and actively incorporate Elder involvement are required to address these gaps.
2. The federal government, First Nations and Métis governments should work in concert to hold national conferences on Aboriginal women and home care, to bring together the various sectors and players to create dialogue and to develop policy directions, research agendas and educational programs that are representative of the various stakeholders needs and visions.
3. Aboriginal home care training needs to be the subject of further research to determine how best to address the unique needs of Aboriginal women students, how best to incorporate Aboriginal culture and languages within the program models, and how best to provide flexible and accessible training models.
4. Research conducted and controlled by Aboriginal people needs to be done to determine to what extent existing training programs are meeting the needs of the communities they serve and enabling service users to stay within their communities. This information can then inform program development and delivery in other Aboriginal communities.

CONCLUSION

In this chapter, we have concentrated on the need for culturally appropriate home care services that reflect the needs and circumstances of Aboriginal women and their communities. As the primary caregivers of home care, both formally and informally, Aboriginal women, and particularly Elders as traditional community leaders, must be at the forefront of envisioning, creating and implementing Aboriginal home care services.

Currently, there are only limited home care services that are culturally congruent and readily accessible to the 689 First Nations, and the numerous Inuit and Métis communities across Canada, all of which have unique and diverse health care needs. Filling this gap is of great concern as the demand for Aboriginal health care services continues to increase. Building community capacity to provide home care services to Aboriginal people must be done in a fashion that respects the diverse traditions and cultures of Aboriginal people. As an extension of Aboriginal culture, home care is a vital part of the well-being of the communities as a whole. All measures possible must therefore be taken to ensure that Aboriginal women are integrally involved in the development and implementation of policies, programs research, and training.

References

Abele, F. (1989). *Gathering Strength*. Calgary: Arctic Institute of North America, University of Calgary.

Anderson, M. and K. Parent. (1999). *Putting a Face on Home Care: CARP's Report on Home Care in Canada 1999*. Kingston: Queen's Health Policy Research Unit.

Armstrong, P., M. Boscoe, B. Clow, K. Grant, A. Pederson, Willson, O. Hankivsky, B. Jackson and M. Morrow. (2003). *Reading Romanow: The Implications of the Final Report of the Commission on the Future of Health Care in Canada for Women*. Toronto: National Co-ordinating Group on Health Care Reform and Women.

Assembly of First Nations (AFN) (2000). *Fact Sheet: Disability*. Ottawa: AFN Communications Unit.

——— Resolution No. 37/99. http://www.afn.ca/resolutions/1999/aga percent20resolutions percent201999/res37.htm

——— (2002). *Housing Fact Sheet*. http://www.afn.ca/Programs/Housing/housing_fact_sheet.htm

Aurora College. (1997). *Program Outline: Home and Community Support Worker*. Northwest Territories.

Bonvillain, N. (2001). *Native Nations: Cultures and Histories of Native North America*. New Jersey: Prentice-Hall Inc.

Brotman, S. (2002). "The Primacy of Family in Elder Care Discourse: Home Care Services to Older Ethnic Women in Canada." *Journal of Gerontological Social Work, 38* (3).

Browne, A., J. Fiske and G. Thomas. (2000). *First Nations Women's Encounters with Mainstream Health Care Services and Systems*. Vancouver: B.C. Centre of Excellence for Women's Health.

Browne, P.L. (2000). *Unsafe Practices: Restructuring and Privatization in Ontario Health Care*. Ottawa: Canadian Centre for Policy Alternatives.

Buchignani, N. and C. Armstrong-Esther. (1999). "Informal Care and Older Native Canadians." *Aging and Society, 19* (i1).

Butot, M., P. Hutton, K.S. Makaroff, C. Vezza, and C. van Mossel. (2002). *The Canadian Continuum of Care Act: A Brief to the Royal Commission on the Future of Health Care in Canada*. Victoria, B.C.: University of Victoria.

Canada. Royal Commission on Aboriginal Peoples. *Report of the Royal Commission on Aboriginal Peoples, volume 3, Gathering Strength*.

——— *Report of the Royal Commission on Aboriginal Peoples, volume 4, Perspectives and Realities.*

Canada Mortgage Housing Corporation. *Research and Development Highlights.* Issue 34. July 1997. Ottawa. Page 3.

Canadian Medical Association. (1994). *Bridging the Gap: Promoting Health and Healing for Aboriginal Peoples in Canada.* Ottawa.

Canadian Women's Health Network. (2003). *Gender and Unpaid Caregiving in Canada.* Retrieved from http://www.cwhn.ca

Congress of Aboriginal Peoples. (1999). *Statistical Comparison Chart.* Retrieved from www.abo-peoples.org

Dickason, O.P. (1992). *Canada's First Nations.* Toronto: McClelland and Stewart Inc.

Drescher, E. (1998). *Calling It Work: Taking Caregiving From the Private to the Public.* Retrieved from http://www.mothersarewomen.com/ci_art5.htm.

Elias, B., A. Leader, D. Sanderson and J. O'Neil. (2000). *Living in Balance: Gender, Structural Inequalities, and Health Promoting Behaviors in Manitoba First Nation Communities.* Winnipeg: Northern Health Research Unit, University of Manitoba.

First Nations and Inuit Health Branch. (2003). *First Nations and Inuit Home and Community Care Program.* Health Canada: Ottawa.

Frideres, J.S. (1998). *Aboriginal Peoples in Canada: Contemporary Conflicts* (5th ed.). Scarborough, Ontario: Prentice Hall Allyn and Bacon Canada.

Grant, A. (1996). *No End of Grief: Indian Residential Schools in Canada.* Winnipeg: Pemmican Publications Inc.

Gregory, D. (1988). "An Exploration of the Contact Between Nurses and Indian Elders/ Traditional Healers on Indian Reserves and Health Centres in Manitoba," in E. Young (ed.), *Health Care Issues in the Canadian North.* Edmonton: Boreal Institute for Northern Studies.

Grey Wolf. (2000). *Native American Wisdom: A Practical and Inspirational Guide.* London: Judy Piatkus (Publishers) Ltd..

Federation of Saskatchewan Indian Nations. (1990) *Home Care on Reserve: A Framework.*

Health Canada. (1994). *National Consultation on Continuing Care Needs in First Nations Communities.* Ottawa: Minister of Health

——— (1999). *How Much Fish and Game is Safe to Eat?* Retrieved from www.canadian-healthnetwork.ca/faq-faq/environmental_health-ante_de_lenvironnement/6e.html.

——— (1999A). *A Second Diagnostic on the Health of First Nations and Inuit People in Canada.* Retrieved from http://www.hc-sc.gc.ca.

——— (1999b). *Do Contaminants in the Environment Affect my Health?* Retrieved from www.canadian-health-network.ca/faq-faq/environmental_health-ante_de_lenvironnement/2e.html.

——— (2000a). *Canada's Seniors: Aboriginal Population.* Retrieved from www.hc-sc.gc.ca/seniors-aines/pubs/factoids/en/no15.htm

——— (2000b). *Final Report: First Nations and Inuit Home Care. Health Transition Fund Proposal NA108.* Ottawa: Minister of Public Works and Government Services Canada.

——— (2001a). *Tobacco Reduction.* Retrieved from http://www.hc-sc.gc.ca/fnihb/cp/annualreview/tobacco_reduction.htm.

——— (2001b). *First Nations and Inuit Home and Community Care Program: Program Criteria.* Retrieved from http://www.hc-sc.gc.ca/fnihb/phcph/fnihccp/program_criteria.htm.

——— (2002a). *The Health of Aboriginal Women.* Retrieved from http://www.hc-sc.gc.ca/english/women/facts_issues/facts_aborig.htm.

——— (2002b). *Fetal Alcohol Syndrome, Fetal Alcohol Effect.* Retrieved from http://www.hc-sc.gc.ca/fnihb/cp/fas_fae/introduction.htm

——— (2002c). *Health Transition Fund Project (NA1012): Diabetes Community /*
Home Support Services for First Nations and Inuit. Ottawa: Health Canada. Retrieved from www.hc-sc.gc.ca/fnihb/phcph/fnihccp/trans_funds/health_transition_fund_na1012.htm

——— (2003). *Educational Institutions Offering Training.* First Nations and Inuit Health Branch. Retrieved from www.hc-sc.gc.ca.

Hennessy, C.H. and R. John. (1996). "American Indian Family Caregivers' Perceptions of Burden and Needed Support Services." *Journal of Applied Gerontology,* 15 (3).

Indian and Northern Affairs Canada. (2002a). *Demographics.* Retrieved from http://www.ainc-inac.gc.ca/gs/dem_e.html.

———— (2002b). *Basic Departmental Data 2001.* Ottawa.

Kwantlen University College. (2003). *Continuing Education.* Retrieved from http://www.kwantlence.com.

Milloy, J.S. (1978). *The Era of Civilization: British Policy for the Indians of Canada 1830-1860.* Oxford: University of Oxford Press.

Morris, M. (2001). *Gender-sensitive Home and Community Care and Caregiving Research: A Synthesis Paper.* Ottawa: Health Canada.

National Aboriginal Health Organization and Commission on the Future of Health Care in Canada. (2002). *Draft Proceedings from Aboriginal Forum on Dialogue on Aboriginal Health: Sharing Our Challenges and Our Successes.* Alymer, Quebec.

Navarro, V. (Ed.). *Imperialism, Health and Medicine: Policy, Politics, Health and Medicine.* New York: Baywood Publishing Company.

O'Neil, J.D. (1988). "Referrals to Traditional Healers: The Role of Medical Interpreters," in E. Young (ed.), *Health Care Issues in the Canadian North.* Edmonton: Boreal Institute for Northern Studies.

Perrone, B., H.H. Stockel and V. Krueger. (1991). *Medicine Women, Curanderas, and Women Doctors.* University of Oklahoma Press: Norman and London.

Petawabano, B.M. (2000). "Planning Research for Greater Community Involvement and Long-term Benefit." *Canadian Medical Association Journal,* 163 (10).

Reading, J. (1999). *An Examination of Residential Schools and Elder Health. In First Nation and Inuit Regional Health Survey.* First Nations and Inuit Regional Health Survey National Steering Committee.

Rhoades, E.R. (2000). *American Indian Health: Innovations in Health Care, Promotion, and Policy.* Baltimore: The Johns Hopkins University Press.

Salt River First Nations. (2003). *Program Report: Our Babies Our Future, Our Kids Our Future.* Fort Smith: Northwest Territories.

Satzewich, V. and T. Wotherspoon. (2000). *First Nations: Race, Class and Gender Relations.* Canada: Houghton Boston.

Siemens, T. (2003). *Aboriginal Home Care: Policy Development and Analysis.* Unpublished paper prepared for SW835: Current Aboriginal Issues in Social Work Practice, University of Regina, Saskatchewan.

Statistics Canada. (2002). *Employment by Industry and sex.* Retrieved from www.statcan.ca.

———— (2003). *Aboriginal People in Canada: A Demographic Profile.*

Status of Women Canada. (2001). *Canadian Experience in Gender Mainstreaming.* Ottawa.

Tobias, J. (1976). "Protection, Civilization, Assimilation: An Outline History of Canada's Indian Policy." *The Western Canadian Journal of Anthropology* 13-20.

Waldram, J.B. (1995). *Aboriginal Health in Canada.* Toronto: Toronto University Press.

Women's Health Policy. (2002). *Gender and Unpaid Caregiving in Canada.* Retrieved from www.cwhn.ca.

Xavier, Cattarinich, N.G. and A.J. Cave. (2001). "Assessing Mental Capacity in Canadian Aboriginal Elders." *Social Science and Medicine,* 53(11):1469(1).

Young, D.E. and L.L. Smith. (1992). *The Involvement of Canadian Native Communities in their Health Care Programs: A Review of the Literature since the 1970s.* Edmonton: Centre for the Cross-Cultural Study of Health and Healing.

Young, T. Kue, O'Neil, D.R. John and Elias Brenda. (1999). *Chronic Diseases. In First Nation and Inuit Regional Health Survey.*

"Just Fed and Watered": Women's Experiences of the Gutting of Home Care in Ontario

Jane Aronson

The intersecting effects of economic restructuring, health care reform and population aging have placed new and heightened demands on the home care sector (Armstrong and Armstrong 1996, 1999). Until relatively recently, home care was concerned largely with the needs of frail elderly people and people with disabilities for long-term assistance at home. Now it is also required to address the medical needs of patients discharged quickly from acute hospitals in order to relieve pressure on dwindling hospital beds and budgets. Home care in Canada is still subject to no national standards and provincial governments have, over time, developed various mixes of public, voluntary and commercial service responses. These mixed economies top up and supplement the care provided by families where the bulk of responsibility for care has always rested. They employ a variety of approaches to rationing resources and determining people's entitlement to care, with priority increasingly given to the medical needs of people recovering from acute illness. Consequently, the entitlement of elderly people and people with disabilities to long-term supportive care (e.g., help with bathing, cleaning, food preparation, household maintenance, social support) is reduced and tightly rationed.

These rapid changes in home care are presented in dominant political discourse as the unavoidable consequences of scarce resources and the self-evident imperatives of containing the costs of hospital care. The changes and their justifications are challenged by a wide range of community groups, advocates and labour organizations concerned about mounting tensions at home care's front lines (see, for example, Anderson and Parent 1999; Canadian Centre for Policy Alternatives 2000; Canadian Pensioners Concerned 1998;

Canadian Union of Public Employees 2000; Meade 1999; Ontario Health Coalition 2001). The groups voice a number of key concerns. First, they call attention to the particular jeopardies resulting from home care's physical location – that is, out of public view, in the privacy of people's own homes. "Behind closed doors" (Care Watch Phoneline 1999) home care's insufficiencies for care recipients and its strains for caregivers are obscured and easier to ignore than, for instance, inadequate or exploitative practices in hospitals, doctors' offices or nursing homes.

Second, they articulate concern that the changes in home care, particularly the withering of long-term, supportive home care, have occurred with remarkably little public debate or transparency (Canadian Centre for Policy Alternatives 2000; Meade 2000). Instead, they have been accomplished through incremental changes in service practices and eligibility criteria within service delivery organizations and so, defined in this way as managerial and technical matters to do with enhancing efficiency, they do not come clearly into the public domain as debatable matters of public policy (Clarke and Newman 1997; Stein 2001).

Third, concerned observers note that supportive home care – sometimes termed preventive or social care – is poorly understood and little valued. Concerned with seemingly ordinary activities of daily life (getting up, going to the toilet, washing, dressing, preparing and eating meals, keepings clothes and surroundings clean) supportive care lies ambiguously at the boundary of the medical and the social (Twigg 2000:107). Its claims to enhance care recipients' well-being are difficult to support as it does not fit tidily into dominant scientific and managerial templates in which "inputs" (treatments, services) are clear and "outcomes" (cure, improved functioning) are easily quantified and measurable (Baldock 1997). Further, the work involved in providing supportive home care is not seen as skilled and, because of its association with women's work and domesticity, it is readily trivialized. Home care thus slips easily to the edge of the health care debate where the interests of the acute and institutional care sectors command much greater legitimacy, visibility and influence.

Finally, observers and analysts of home care underscore the reality that its mounting tensions are borne disproportionately by women (Armstrong et al. 2002; Aronson and Neysmith 1997). Women represent the majority of unpaid care providers and are heavily implicated by home care's retreat as it is they who step in to substitute for diminished public care for their relatives even more than before. Women also represent the majority of paid care providers employed in home care: nurses, physiotherapists, occupational therapists, social workers and, numerically the largest group of all, home support workers (variously termed home support/personal support/home care workers). And, last, women form the majority of home care recipients, especially in older age groups.

This chapter aims to illuminate this last group's experiences of the obscured retreat of public home care. In order to do so, I draw on material from a qualitative study of elderly women and women with disabilities who were receiving home care in Ontario between 1998 and 2002. The longitudinal study was based on a sample of twenty-seven women, twenty of them elderly, living with a range of chronic conditions and disabilities. Located through community groups concerned with seniors issues or disabilities, the participants all lived in urban southern Ontario and were distributed through the catchment areas of seven Community Care Access Centres (see below). In successive interviews over three and a half years, the women spoke about their health, their social circumstances and their home care, as well as their histories, joys, worries and aspirations.

The study spanned a period of rapid reorganization and retrenchment in health and home care in Ontario. The province's experience may be particular in that the conservative government in power since 1995 has pursued its ideological commitment to smaller government with exceptional zeal. However, the structuring of home care in all provinces is driven by a central concern to relieve acute hospitals, rather than by a central concern to address the ongoing needs of elderly people and people with disabilities. The experiences of women receiving home care in Ontario will therefore have much in common with those of their counterparts in other provinces and can enhance our understanding of the front-line implications of government retreat from supportive home care provision.

HOME CARE AND THE ONTARIO CONTEXT

Home care is not included in the Canada Health Act and has never been mandated federally as a universal program. However, in the 1960s and 1970s, its development was stimulated by permissive federal-provincial cost-sharing arrangements. Under these provisions, the provinces fashioned a range of approaches to home care, generally building rather fragmented networks of public and voluntary services. However, with the federal government's cuts in transfer payments and a move to block funding in 1995, home care became a matter of almost entirely provincial jurisdiction (Armstrong 2002). At the time of writing, federal and provincial governments are beginning to take up and debate the Romanow Commission's (Commission on the Future of Health Care in Canada 2002) recommendations on home care. The Commission recommended greater federal involvement and initiative, proposing specifically a national platform for home care in selected areas (acute care, palliative care, mental health). Supportive home care was not given the same priority. Instead, the Commission urged that the provinces expand supportive home care "as resources permit" (Commission on the Future of Health Care in Canada 2002:187) . This relatively weak and permissive recommendation, a disappointment to many advocates and community groups, thus leaves supportive home care to the discretion of the provinces.

In Ontario in 1996, the government introduced a market-modelled system of "managed competition" in home care, claiming that it would enhance consumer choice and efficiency (Williams et al. 1999). This approach to home care was part of the government's wider agenda to reduce social spending and, to that end, to frame health and social issues as individual concerns requiring private solutions rather than as collective concerns requiring public solutions. Under managed competition, the role of government is confined to the contracting out of service provision to competing nonprofit and for-profit home care providers and the screening of clients. Forty-three Community Care Access Centres (CCACs) were established across the province to administer the competitive bidding and contracting out process, and to employ case managers to assess individual home care clients' eligibility and coordinate packages of services from contracted providers.

The CCACs faced mounting demand for their services as the Health Services Restructuring Commission, also set up in the government's first term, recommended hospital closures and the downloading of care to people's homes (Armstrong and Armstrong 1999; Gustafson 2000). The transfer of resources expected to accompany this shift in the site of care was not forthcoming. The CCACs scrambled to devise local mechanisms for allocating their services until, in 1999, province-wide regulations were introduced to standardize the rationing of home care (Government of Ontario 1999). These regulations gave priority to the "medically necessary" services required by growing numbers of acute or sub-acute patients being discharged quickly from hospitals to their own homes. As a result, elderly people and people with disabilities in need of long-term supportive care at home were accorded progressively lower priority for service.

Since 1996, the CCACs across the province have been charged with implementing local care markets and competitive contract processes, dealing with mounting demands from the hospital sector, implementing rationing regulations and gauging the particular needs in their local catchment areas – all within capped and unpredictable budgets. Unsurprisingly, they have been sorely challenged to accomplish this mandate. The CCAC in the Hamilton area (where I am located and therefore best acquainted with the dynamics of service organizations) provides an illuminating example of the working-out of these challenges at the local level. The Hamilton CCAC was the focus of controversy and local media attention from 1999 onwards as it over-ran its budget and experienced considerable internal conflict and instability. Characterizing the problems as matters of internal administrative incompetence, the Ministry of Health and Long-Term Care intervened in 2001 by disbanding the voluntary board of directors and appointing a supervisor to take over management of the organization. In doing so, the government modelled its expectations for CCACs in the rest of the province. Charged with containing costs, the Hamilton supervisor oversaw the withdrawal of service from 3,500 clients (of a total caseload of 11,000) most of whom had been receiving ongoing supportive forms of care. The supervisor explained: "We can't keep people on for life. The hospital will discharge you and home care does the same thing" (Dumanian 2002). In support of her actions, the Associate Minister of Health and Long-Term Care at that time asserted an apparently self-evident distinction between medical care and supportive social care in a reminder that the government priority was not cleaning people's houses: "I remind people that this is the Ministry of Health funding these services and our major objective is to provide health services" (Johns 2002).

Soon afterwards, the government introduced legislation to convert the CCACs to statutory corporations with government-appointed executive directors and boards of directors. A key channel for democratic debate and local input was thus eliminated. Debate did continue in the local media in Hamilton as concerned citizens and advocates kept calling attention to the damaging implications of cutting supportive care. Pressed on this point, the chair of the new government-appointed CCAC board expressed satisfaction that "the books are balanced and the CCAC is doing a better job of abiding by the province's stringent new rules about who qualifies for home care. I'm feeling good about what we're doing as an agency. We're following the guidelines to a 't'" (Mullan 2002).

Hamilton's experiences of the government's changes in home care are paralleled throughout the province and have been well charted by organizations like the Ontario Health Coalition and the Ontario Coalition of Senior Citizens' Organizations. Supportive, long-term home care is articulated as a discretionary extra, secondary to the CCACs' central focus on medical care. And, as is evident from Mullan's quote, compliance with government direction and managerial efficiency are given primacy, without reference to questions of unmet need and the implications of withdrawing supportive care.

To explore these implications from care recipients' perspectives, the story of one study participant, Mrs. X, offers an illuminating entry point.

Mrs. X

When I first met Mrs. X in 1998, she was 79 and had been a widow for almost ten years. She lived alone in an apartment in the Toronto area. Despite the mounting constraints of arthritis and a heart condition, she felt fairly optimistic that she would be able to stay there – her dearest wish. She had begun receiving help at home five years before and, at the time we met, was considered by her local CCAC to be eligible for three visits (three hours each) per week from a home support worker. This worker helped her with bathing, household tasks (light cleaning, laundry, cooking) and exercises, and would occasionally walk with her the short block to her bank and a corner store. Besides accomplishing needed errands, the exercise was good for her and she benefited from the outing: "I like to see what's happening in the street and let them know I'm still here!" she told me robustly. Mrs. X was also considered eligible for a monthly nursing visit to monitor her medications and check on her overall health: "I feel more confident with her (the nurse) knowing how I am; she's known me a long time and we talk about everything really .. how I'm eating and how to avoid falling, all that sort of thing." Mrs. X managed her shopping through a combination of a supermarket delivery service and the help of her older daughter who lives about an hour's drive away.

A few months after our first meeting, Mrs. X's case manager informed her that her services would have to be reduced because the CCAC was facing severe budget cuts: "She said they have to see people who are ill, not people like me who just need a bit of help to manage." Accordingly, Mrs. X's nurse's visit was eliminated and her home support worker's allotted time cut from three visits to two shorter visits a week. For a time, the nurse tried to stay in touch with her by telephone and was a reassuring presence: "It was so kind of her, we'd become friends but she couldn't keep it up, I understand that." Mrs. X also struggled to accommodate the reduced home support hours by doing more cleaning herself: "I try to take things slowly, not do anything stupid and be really careful. My daughter worries, I know, but I hate not feeling tidy and at home. I don't want people to think I'm letting things go."

One year later, Mrs. X's support worker's hours were reduced again, this time to a single one-hour visit per week, exclusively for the purpose of giving her a bath. Mrs. X asked the worker if she could pay her privately to come a second time each week: "She said she'd like to, but they're not allowed to do it. It's too bad, I like her and you don't want someone you don't know in, do you? ... especially not helping you in the bathroom?" Since that time, Mrs. X's home support worker has changed numerous times. The nonprofit agency to whose worker she had been accustomed lost its contract with her CCAC. Mrs. X was first reassigned to another nonprofit and then to a for-profit agency. Both organizations were unable to provide consistent workers.

This instability and reduction in services has distressed and drained Mrs. X enormously. She feels "humiliated" at her poor hygiene and at the untidy state of her apartment. She seldom goes out, seldom asks anyone in and her appetite is poor. She is falling more, sometimes while attempting tasks that strain her physical capacity (taking a sponge bath, cooking, doing laundry by hand). Her daughter tries to come more often but: "It's such a long drive for her and she works hard and when she's here we don't really have a visit, she just gets me sorted out until the next time. I'm just a drag on her now." Reluctantly, Mrs. X allows her other daughter, who lives out of province, to cover extra expenses like the cost of grocery and pharmacy deliveries and occasional house cleaning. To accomplish the latter, Mrs. X put an advertisement in her local corner store window but felt uncertain of the person who responded: "She seemed nosy about what I'd got here, it made me nervous and I didn't ask her back." She resorted, instead, to a cleaning service: "But it's much more expensive and neither of my girls (daughters) have money to spare and I've no extra so I try not to have them in often. But look at the place ..."

Four years after our first interview, and in accordance with government policy, Mrs. X's home care had been radically reduced. However, she finds no fault with the individual service providers she sees. Of the home support workers, she says: "The girls are so rushed, they never know what their next week's work looks like, they don't have it easy." And of her CCAC case manager: "It can't be much fun telling people what they can't have all the time, can it? So I don't make any fuss, I don't want to make it harder for her." Mrs. X notes also that she would never complain because: "I don't want to get known as a troublemaker, especially not now. I've just got to learn to manage on my own and I must be grateful."

Mrs. X now anticipates that she will have to "give up" but "dreads" the prospect of a nursing home: "I used to enjoy life; now I'm really just waiting for the bone yard." At our final meeting in 2002 she reflected: "I thought they wanted to keep people all right in their own homes, they said they did. But they seem to want to keep me just fed and watered here – that's all."

Mrs. X is a single instance, a "case," but her experience of home care over several years reveals how it is shrinking and being shifted out of the public domain. Her experience gives us a glimpse, too, at the reverberations for her sense of self, her identity and spirit generated by public policy retreat in home care. These two themes are elaborated below, substantiated at times by the accounts of other study participants.

SHIFTING AND PRIVATIZING THE WORK AND RESPONSIBILITY OF CARE

In Mrs. X's account, we can discern the everyday, incremental processes through which home care is being offloaded from the public arena. To conceptualize and map this easily obscured process, Szebehely (1998) generated a typology to capture the possible combinations of funding and provision of care and the "trends toward informalization and marketization." A slightly adapted version of this typology, presented below, illuminates the shift of publicly funded and publicly provided care to other social contexts and relationships.

WHO PROVIDES THE CARE?

Who pays?	Family	State	Market	Voluntary Sector
Care work unpaid	1a	2a	3a	4a
Care work publicly financed	1b	2b	3b	4b
Care work privately financed within formal economy	1c	2c	3c	4c
Care work privately financed within informal economy	1d	2d	3d	4d

Like all typologies, the categories risk rigidifying and simplifying com-plexities and require qualification in places. For example, the offloading of public responsibility for home care is depicted as the dispersal of care outwards from cell 2b, publicly financed and publicly provided care. In the past, in Ontario and most other provinces, publicly financed care was not delivered exclusively by public sector, state-employed providers but was also delegated to voluntary, nonprofit organizations (e.g., the Victorian Order of Nurses and the Red Cross) and so was a blurred combination of cells 2b and 4b. Now, under managed competition, no publicly financed care is publicly provided. Instead it is contracted out on a competitive basis to a mix of nonprofit and for-profit providers (cells 3b and 4b) and case management is the only function still performed by publicly paid employees (cell 2b). With this clarification, however, Szebehely's (1998) typology offers a helpful conceptual map in which to locate and make sense of the experiences of people like Mrs. X.

OFFLOADING CARE FROM THE PUBLIC ARENA (CELL 2B)

Mrs. X experienced the offloading of publicly supported care in her encounters with her CCAC case manager. Case managers are charged with implementing eligibility criteria at home care's front line. Gatekeepers to home care, they carry a tense combination of responsibilities for both assessing need and rationing resources, for "telling people what they can't have" as Mrs. X put it (Aronson and Sinding 2000). Mrs. X's case manager gradually reduced her support to a weekly bath, the norm specified in provincial regulations. The assistance Mrs. X had received previously with cleaning, more frequent bathing and getting out of the house had enabled her to maintain her home and her person in ways she valued. Symbolically, this practical help had supported her sense of self as a social being – as someone still connected to her neighbourhood and who asked visitors into her home. Many study participants shared Mrs. X's distress at the deterioration of their homes and their appearances: "I'm so embarrassed, just look at the place," "I'd be ashamed to have anyone here now – it's not *me*, you know, I've never lived like this." Effectively, the stripping away of supportive help rendered them little more than dysfunctional bodies, deemed worthy of maintaining only at a minimal level of cleanliness or, in Mrs. X's reduced terms: "just fed and watered."

In addition to the minimalism of her allocation of care, Mrs. X was also troubled by the inconsistency of the personnel who provided it – a concern voiced by most study participants. They found changing care providers both exhausting and intrusive. A younger participant who needed daily help with personal care voiced her frustration and the indignity of her exposure: "You have these strangers coming in and looking after you in very personal places – and you have no choice."

These front-line experiences of inconsistent care workers reflect both the heightening of long-standing problems in underfunded home care organization and new disruptions resulting from the introduction of managed competition. Continuity of care and personnel, known to be a key ingredient in service quality

(Brechin 1998) has always been difficult to provide because of the costs of attention to scheduling and matching, and the difficulty of keeping skilled staff in the face of chronically poor employment conditions. The challenges have, however, been exacerbated because, to stay competitive and win CCAC contracts, provider organizations have been pressed to drive down costs wherever possible (Armstrong and Armstrong 1999; O'Connor, in press). Labour costs are their principal outlay so employment conditions (wage rates, security, benefits, compensation for travel costs and time) have deteriorated and, unsurprisingly, staff retention has suffered. In her sympathetic observation that her workers were "rushed" and on unpredictable schedules, we hear Mrs. X's experience of the front-line manifestations of this turbulence in home care work. She herself made no distinction between workers from nonprofit (cell 3b) or for-profit (cell 4b) agencies. A younger participant reflected more directly and with exasperation: "I don't care where they come from any more – if they'd just be consistent and know what they're doing." Arguably, however, the degradation of employment conditions will be especially marked in the for-profit sector where few workers are unionized and where supportive organizational infrastructures are least developed (Canadian Union of Public Employees 2000).

Despite the distress caused by cuts to her home care and the strain of ever-changing care providers, Mrs. X described her encounters with her case manager fatalistically; indeed, with some sympathy for her position. On the other hand, some study participants voiced anger at their mounting disentitlement to their case managers. For example, a younger woman raged at the application of the weekly bath ration: "Did you know the government's rule is that anyone with a CCAC needs a bath only once a week? I asked her (the case manager) would *she* be content with that? Would anyone in government have a bath once a week?" A few asked their case managers if they could make sure their workers were more consistent. While their requests and distress were sympathetically heard, they were told that little could be done as all contracted provider agencies had similar problems. Significantly, few participants sustained or formalized complaints even if they harboured indignation or criticism. Like Mrs. X who did not want to get known as a "troublemaker," they recognized their jeopardy: "You can't bite the hand that feeds you, you know;" "It could make it worse for me up the road. You have to be careful."

Faced with progressively less public support, participants recognized that they would have to find their own solutions to the challenges they faced in living at home. Like Mrs. X, many resolved stoically to "manage" – an often-used word, loaded with images of endurance and tenacity and, especially among older women, with references to coping with hardships earlier in their lives. They saw themselves as "on their own" – the intended result of public policies that force individual, not collective, solutions to people's needs. Pressed out of the public arena, then, care recipients had to turn to other resources to get their needs met, a shift depicted in Szebehly's (1998) typology by the arrows dispersing care out of cell 2c.

Care Offloaded to Families (Cell 1a)

As is now well recognized, most practical and emotional care occurs in the context of families and is provided predominantly by women (Aronson and Neysmith 1997). Mrs. X's experience reflects this broader distribution of care and highlights, too, the limits to families' resources. To supplement her shrinking allocation of home care and respond to her increasing frailty, Mrs. X's daughters stepped in to the extent that they could, helping with cleaning and shopping and offsetting the costs of buying such help privately. As Mrs. X's case manager reduced her services, she explicitly suggested that Mrs. X's daughter come more often and help her around the house. Other participants reported similar exchanges and suggestions. Such suggestions are based on unspoken assumptions about family relationships and are probably intended to help home care clients manage the withdrawal of public care. In effect, though, these encounters and their assumptions exact from care recipients' relatives (usually women) what has been termed "enforced altruism" and shift the boundary between public entitlement and private responsibility (Davis and Ellis 1995).

Mrs. X, in company with other study participants and with older people described in the literature, was reluctant to accept help from her daughters (Aronson 1990; Daatland 1990). She sadly described how visits with her daughter that had once been enjoyable and reciprocal social occasions had become simply work for her daughter and troubling for her. She felt herself "just a drag on her now." She and others identified the already strained lives of the relatives on whom they were forced to depend. For example, an older participant was reticent to further "burden" a daughter who held down two part-time jobs organized around the care of a child with a developmental disability; a woman in her 50s noted that she could not keep looking to her mother for help: "She's in her 80s now; she can't be running up and down after me." The dependence on family and informal sources enforced by home care's retreat should not, then, be understood as welcomed or simple.

A number of study participants described situations where such an understanding was particularly problematic and misplaced. With cuts to her home care, an older woman had to turn to a daughter with whom she had a troubled relationship and of whom she felt afraid. As has long been pointed out, the possibilities of abuse and harm within families are heightened when relatives are coerced into caring by the absence of outside supports (Neysmith 1995). Several participants described the inappropriateness of case managers' efforts to transfer responsibilities to neighbours and friends. For example, a participant in her 50s resented being told that, because the home support agency that supplied her workers was short-staffed over a holiday weekend, she should ask the parish nurse at her church to help her up in the morning and to bed at night: "They'd no right! We don't have that kind of relationship. She's a kind person, but I'm very private and she shouldn't have to!" Finally, of course, assumptions about simply transferring care to the unpaid hands of families, friends and neighbours break down entirely for people who are isolated or have limited social networks – the harsh reality for several of this study's participants.

Care Offloaded to the Marketplace (Cells 3c and 3d)

Study participants who could afford to do so purchased a range of services to sustain and expand their living at home (e.g., cleaning services, home deliveries, accompaniment to appointments or outside activities, take-out meals). Szebehely (1998) makes an important distinction between care privately purchased in the formal economy (cell 3c) and care privately purchased in the informal or grey economy (cell 3d). Mrs. X engaged in the former when, for example, she paid a commercial company for house cleaning. Some participants reported that their case managers facilitated such arrangements to maintain their hours of home care service. For example: "She (case manager) told me she had to cut the girl's hours down to two but, if I wanted to pay privately for the other two – so I kept the help with cooking – then I could." Accordingly, two hours of this participant's home support worker were covered by the CCAC and she paid the contracted nonprofit agency directly for her other two hours. In this way, she kept a worker with whom she was familiar and whom she liked.

Some study participants also sought assistance in the informal economy. Mrs. X, for instance, began her search for extra cleaning help through her neighbourhood store; another woman pinned up an ad in her apartment building laundry room. The person that Mrs. X located was much cheaper than the commercial cleaning service to which she eventually turned. However, the uncertainty surrounding such informal arrangements discomfited her and some other participants: "You never know who you're getting do you?;" "I'm not that pleased with the help but you can't say much ... I don't know how else to find help I can afford."

Requesting reassurance that I would tell no one, another older woman described how she had successfully worked out an agreement "under the table" with a CCAC-financed worker whose hours had been cut: "She comes on the weekend and gives me another bath and tidies up. It works OK for us both. She gets a bit extra and I know I can trust her. Of course, we keep it very quiet – it's against all the rules." This particular arrangement, rooted in familiarity, worked well but there is evident potential for tension and vulnerability in care relations negotiated in this informal marketplace. For example, a participant in her 60s described her anxiety and sense of vulnerability when she accused a personal care worker whom she had located through a local newspaper of stealing from her; and an older participant attributed her cleaner's "sloppiness" to her cultural background. Such encounters highlight the possibilities of disempowerment and discrimination for both recipients and providers of assistance who come to such relationships with few resources, few options and no recourse or protection if things go badly (Neysmith and Aronson 1997; Ungerson 1999).

Market solutions to care needs are, of course, much heralded by neo-liberal governments eager to characterize care recipients as consumers with choices to exercise. However, just as unpaid family care is not a resort for people without available families, so market solutions to insufficient home care are not a resort for people who cannot pay for them. Of the twenty-seven participants in this study, eleven were poor and therefore quite unable to engage in either formal or informal economies. This figure mirrors the population-based proportions of elderly women and women with disabilities who live only on government transfers and are poor or near-poor (National Council on Welfare 1997).

Care Offloaded to "Conscripted Volunteers" (Cells 3a and 4a)

Care offloaded from the public domain was sometimes taken up, albeit in relatively small ways, by paid care providers who volunteered their time and skills over and above that required by the conditions of their employment. For example, Mrs. X described the continuing support she derived from a visiting nurse after her paid services had been withdrawn by the CCAC. Several other participants reported similar ways in which paid care providers extended themselves to help them by providing some of the assistance that had been formally cut off (e.g., bringing shopping round, washing hair, cutting toenails, visiting to lessen their isolation). Such instances of rule-breaking and "going beyond the call of duty" are noted in the small literature on home care work (e.g., Aronson and Neysmith 1996). Little is known about them as they transgress the boundaries of employment conditions and professionalism and are, therefore, kept quiet. Indeed, study participants occasionally reminded me that they must stay shrouded: "Now, I'm telling you but the case manager mustn't know or we'd both (herself and her home care worker) be in trouble."

While often described as warming acts of kindness and generosity, these extensions of paid caring roles require the time and energy of workers and are prompted by concern – borne in isolation – about vulnerable and isolated home care recipients. It is unclear, therefore, whether they can be considered truly voluntary activities.

CARE OFFLOADED TO RECIPIENTS THEMSELVES

In describing her efforts to manage at home, Mrs. X revealed a variety of ways in which she tried herself to take up the slack left by cuts to her home care. For example, she struggled to keep her apartment as "presentable" as she could and, with laborious sponge baths, to sustain her standards of personal hygiene. Study participants exerted enormous efforts to care for themselves and absorb the impacts of reduced home care help – efforts that fly in the face of the dominant characterization of care recipients as passive, non-contributors to care (Barry 1995). Their labour – in all its physical, emotional, moral and political dimensions – has been poorly captured in theoretical analyses of care. Its illumination in study participants' accounts is, therefore, particularly valuable and suggests the importance of adding a fifth column to Szebehely's (1998) typology: "the care recipient."

The physical dimensions and costs of participants' efforts to accommodate the withdrawal of home care are well-represented in Mrs. X's account. She and other participants engaged in creative and tenacious strategies to sustain themselves in as acceptable and dignified a manner as they could. One participant with very limited mobility, and who used a wheelchair most of the time, described how she managed to wash her hair at the kitchen sink – a complicated and exhausting activity, but one that made her feel "more human." She knew it was also a very precarious activity, just as Mrs. X knew she ran more risks of falling as she tried to do small household tasks. Significantly, when I invited participants to tell me about the details of these determined labours, they generally dismissed their significance. For instance, of the hair washing: "You don't want to know about that do you? (Yes …) Well, I can't think it's of much interest to anyone … I've never really thought about it or put it into words … you just do it." Obscured from our cultural and analytical view as domestic and trivial, these dogged labours and acts of resistance were, unsurprisingly, obscured from participants' view too.

Participants also engaged in "the work of shaping needs to available care provision" (Barry 1995:372) reducing themselves to match the reductions in their home care. Thus, for instance, Mrs. X stopped inviting people to her apartment. She discouraged a neighbour who used to drop in and told her few remaining friends that she preferred to keep in touch by phone. Without an audience, her need to be "presentable" and "respectable" was less and she could let go of past standards of housekeeping and appearance. Another older woman gradually concentrated her activities and her life into her bedroom; she could no longer keep up the rest of the house and closed rooms off so that she would not have to see them. Giving up cooking or preparing appetizing meals was another common accommodation. While often reluctantly made, it was simpler than struggling to manage shopping and cooking against insurmountable odds – odds heightened for those who had neither family members nor the financial means to beat them.

Home care's retreat also required study participants to exercise different "practices of care reception" (Barry 1995:372). For example, in response to home care cuts, Mrs. X strove to negotiate different solutions to her needs, initially with her familiar home care worker and, later, with a cleaner and a commercial cleaning service. Some participants engaged more actively with care providers in efforts to better adapt care to their particular needs. For example, a few women sought to change the time or day on which their bath was scheduled; and several strove to adapt their home care workers' assignments to their preferences, for example, to help with laundry rather than with tidying the bathroom. Participants clearly gave thought to the most productive and least jeopardizing ways of making these demands and conducting their negotiations. As we have seen, most judged it wise to strike an uncomplaining posture; despite the shortcomings of their care, they muted complaint and often voiced gratitude for what they received.

Just as family, marketplace and voluntary solutions to home care users' unmet needs are inequitably distributed so, too, are their capacities to engage in the physical, cognitive and political work of receiving and accommodating themselves to insufficient care. For people with severe physical impairments, assuming more household and personal care tasks is simply not practically possible. Negotiating with public and commercial service providers requires interpersonal and bureaucratic skills. These capacities are typically associated with social class and cultural capital and the study sample offered some glimpses at the inequities and barriers these divisions generated. For example, a younger participant who termed herself obese felt that service providers were scornful of her and dismissed her needs. An older woman reflected that she knew she should not "talk back" to her case manager: "but I don't have the gift of the gab, not like some people who can be "oh so polite" and get people to like them ... I never learned that, not the way I was raised." The sample of experience in this study encompassed differences in class, age and ability; research that captures greater variation in social locations, particularly, race and culture is needed. However, the knowledge we do have strongly and unsurprisingly suggests that "those who have traditionally been most vulnerable are facing deteriorating conditions of care" (Armstrong 2002:308).

CONCLUSION

The experiences of women receiving care at home have been discussed here to explore the implications for them of the hollowing out of supportive home care. Seldom included as knowledgeable participants in policy discussions, the perspectives of these women reveal the privately borne human and economic costs of the retreat of public home care. They also offer important glimpses at the potential jeopardy of differently located paid and unpaid care providers. Care is most accurately understood as a relationship. Thus, the experiences of both its recipients and its providers require attention in efforts to support it and ensure its quality. The questions articulated by Armstrong and Kits in Chapter 2 to assess care-related legislation, regulations and policy can be usefully asked of all the relations and sites of care discussed here and mapped by Szebehely (1998) in order to discern their fairness, safety, respectfulness of the interests of receivers and providers, and short-and long-term consequences.

The experiences of women like those introduced here also underscore the shortsightedness of the economic arguments underlying the current direction of provincial home care policies. Specifically, the claim that supportive assistance with personal care and the maintenance of a home are of little relevance to people's health and well-being (and can, thus, be easily withdrawn) is clearly flawed. To return to Mrs. X as an illustrative case, the withdrawal of public support for a presentable home, a presentable appearance and connection to her social surroundings clearly undermined her self-respect and her health. It is highly likely that her crushed spirit and overtaxed personal resources will generate the health care costs that come with falls, physical depletion and depression. This shortsighted approach to rationing and targeting home care runs counter to the evidence of these long-term costs and consequences that is gradually accumulating in a variety of jurisdictions (e.g., Clark 2001; Clark et al. 1998; Dalley 1998, 2001; Hollander and Chappell 2002; Pollak 2000; Thorslund 1997; Wistow and Hardy 1999). In the short term, some modest costs may be saved in this way. Generated in the long term, though, are economic costs, as well as distress and heightened social inequities.

As provincial and federal governments begin to discuss the recommendations of the Romanow Commission (Commission on the Future of Health Care in Canada 2002) and future directions in home care, it will be crucial to intrude this kind of evidence into debate. Looking beyond health care and the strategic opportunity that the Commission has presented, it is also important that the experiences of people like Mrs. X be understood more broadly. Elderly people and people with disabilities are not just ill-served health and home care users. They are citizens excluded from full social participation. "Just fed and watered," they are contained out of public view in the isolation of their own homes. Their exclusion can be more fully understood as a denial of human rights – a framing that may suggest additional directions for action and research and the potential for building common cause with other groups unjustly deprived of their social citizenship by a retreating state.

We gratefully acknowledge the participants in the study for sharing their knowledge and time. A number of community groups provided useful links and have been supportive of the project in an ongoing way. Their input is much appreciated – in particular, the help of Mae Harman of Canadian Pensioners Concerned and Ethel Meade of the Older Women's Network. The work reported here is supported by research grants from the Social Sciences and Humanities Research Council (Women and Change #816-98-0042) and the National Network on Environments and Women's Health (a Centre of Excellence in Women's Health funded by the Women's Health Bureau of Health Canada).

References

Anderson, M. and K. Parent. (1999). *Putting a Face on Home Care: CARP's Report on Home Care in Canada 1999*. Kingston: Queen's Health Policy Research Unit.

Armstrong, P. (2002). "The Context of Health Care Reform in Canada.," p. 11-48 in P. Armstrong et al. (eds.), *Exposing Privatization: Women and Health Reform in Canada*. Aurora: Garamond.

Armstrong, P., C. Amaratunga, J. Bernier, K. Grant, A. Pederson and K. Willson (eds.). (2002). *Exposing Privatization: Women and Health Reform in Canada*. Aurora: Garamond.

Armstrong, P. and H. Armstrong. (1996). *Wasting Away: The Undermining of Canadian Health Care*. Toronto: Oxford University Press.

————— (1999). *Women, Privatization and Health Care Reform: The Ontario Scan*. Toronto: National Network on Environments and Women's Health, York University.

Aronson, J. (1990). "Old Women's Experiences of Needing Care: Choice or Compulsion?" *Canadian Journal on Aging*, 9 (3): 234-247.

————— (2002). "Frail and Disabled Users of Home Care: Confident Consumers or Disentitled Citizens?" *Canadian Journal on Aging* 21 (1): 11-26.

Aronson, J. and S.M. Neysmith. (1996). "'You're Not Just in There to do the Work': Depersonalizing Policies and the Exploitation of Home Care Workers' Labour." *Gender and Society*, 10, 59-77.

————— (1997). "The Retreat of the State & Long-Term Care Provision: Implications for Frail Elderly People, Unpaid Family Carers & Paid Home Care Workers." *Studies in Political Economy*, 53: 37-66.

————— (2001). "Manufacturing Social Exclusion in the Home Care Market." *Canadian Public Policy*, XXVII, 151-165.

Aronson, J. and C. Sinding. (2000). "Home Care Users' Experiences of Fiscal Constraints: Challenges and Opportunities for Case Management." *Care Management Journals* 2 (4): 1-6.

Baldock, J. (1997). "Social Care in Old Age: More Than a Funding Problem." *Social Policy and Administration*, 31, 73-89.

Barry, J. (1995). "Care-need and Care-receivers: Views From the Margins." *Women's Studies International Forum*, 18, 351-374.

Brechin, A. (1998). "What Makes for Good Care?" p. 17-186 in A. Brechin et al. (eds.), *Care Matters: Concepts, Practice and Research in Health and Social Care*. London: Sage.

Canadian Centre for Policy Alternatives. (2000). *Without Foundation: How Medicare is Undermined by Gaps and Privatization in Community and Continuing Care*. Vancouver: CCPA.

Canadian Pensioners Concerned, Ontario Division. (1998). *Position Statement on Privatization in Health Care*. Toronto.

Canadian Union of Public Employees. (2000). *Who's Pushing Privatization? Annual Report on Privatization*. Ottawa: CUPE.

Care Watch Phone Line. (1999). *Behind Closed Doors: Home Care Stories from the Community*. Toronto: Care Watch Toronto.

Clark, J. (2001). "Preventive Home Visits to Elderly People: Their Effectiveness Cannot be Judged by Randomized Control Trials." *British Medical Journal* 323, p.708.

Clark, H., S. Dyer and J. Horwood. (1998). *That Bit of Help: The High Value of Low Level Preventative Services for Older People*. Bristol: Policy Press.

Clarke, J. and J. Newman. (1997). *The Managerial State*. London: Sage.

Commission on the Future of Health Care in Canada. (2002). *Building on Values: The Future of Health Care in Canada*. Ottawa.

Daatland, S. (1990). "What Are Families For? On Family Solidarity and Preference for Help." *Aging and Society* 10.

Dalley, G. (1998). *Defining Difference: Health and Social Care for Older People in the 1990s*. London: Centre for Policy on Aging.

Dalley, G. 2001. *The Passive Privatisation of Social Welfare Services for Older People in the U.K.* Paper presented at the 17th World Congress of the International Association of Gerontology, Vancouver.

Davis, A. and K. Ellis. (1995). "Enforced Altruism in Community Care," p.136-154 in R. Hugman and D. Smith (eds.), *Ethical Issues in Social Work.* London: Routledge.

Dumanian, J. (2002). Quoted in *Hamilton Spectator*, 15 February, p. A8.

Government of Ontario (1999). *Provision of Community Services. Ontario Regulation 386/99 Made Under the Long Term Care Act 1994.* Toronto: Gazette of Ontario.

Gustafson, D. (2000). "Home Care Before and After Reform: A Comparative Analysis of Two Texts in Action," p. 177- 198 in D. Gustafson (ed.), *Care and Consequences: The Impact of Health Care Reform.* Halifax: Fernwood.

Hollander, M. and N. Chappell. (2002). *Final Report of the National Evaluation of the Cost-Effectiveness of Home Care.* Victoria: Centre on Aging.

Johns, H. (2002). Quoted in *Hamilton Spectator*, 15 February, p. A8.

Meade, E. (1999). "Health Care Issues." *Older Women's Network: Contact* 11 (2): 4.

—— (2000). "Will the Public be Consulted About the New Long-term Care Act?" *Older Women's Network: Contact* 12 (3), 5.

Mullan, B. (2002). Quoted in *Hamilton Spectator*, 31 July, A8.

National Council of Welfare. (1997). *Poverty Profile 1995.* Ottawa: Ministry of Supply and Services.

Neysmith, S.M. (1995). "Power in Relationships of Trust: A Feminist Analysis of Elder Abuse," p. 43-54 in M. MacLean (ed.), *Abuse and Neglect of Older Canadians: Strategies for Change.* Toronto: Thompson Educational Publishing.

Neysmith, S.M. and J. Aronson. (1997). "Working Conditions in Home Care: Negotiating Race & Class Boundaries in Gendered Work." *International Journal of Health Services*, 27 (3): 479-499.

O'Connor, D. (in press). "Offloading the Cost of Home Care: The Impacts on Front Line Workers and Agencies," in P. Leduc Brown (ed.), *The Commodity of Care: Assessing Ontario's Experiment with Managed Competition in Home Care.* Ottawa: Canadian Centre for Policy Alternatives.

Ontario Health Coalition. (2001). *Long Term Care – In Limbo or Worse?* Toronto.

Pollak, N. (2000). "Cutting Home Support: From 'Closer to Home' to 'All Alone,'" p. 93 in *Without Foundation: How Medicare is Undermined by Gaps and Privatization in Community and Continuing Care.* Vancouver: Centre for Policy Alternatives.

Stein, J.G. (2001). *The Cult of Efficiency.* Toronto: Anansi Press.

Szebehely, M. (1998). "Concepts and Trends in Home Care for Frail Elderly People in France and Sweden." Conference presentation, *Comparing Social Welfare in Nordic Countries and France.* Paris.

Thorslund, M., A. Bergmark and M.G. Parker. (1997). "Difficult Decisions on Care and Services for Elderly People: The Dilemma of Setting Priorities in the Welfare State." *Scandinavian Journal of Social Welfare* 6: 197-206.

Twigg, J. (2000). *Bathing – The Body and Community Care.* Routledge: London.

Ungerson, C. (1999). "Personal Assistants and Disabled People: An Examination of a Hybrid Form of Work and Care." *Work, Employment and Society* 13 (4): 583-600.

Williams, A.P., J. Barnsley, S. Leggat, R. Deber and P. Baranek. (1999). "Long-term Care Goes to Market: Managed Competition and Ontario's Reform of Community-based Services." *Canadian Journal on Aging,* 18, 125-153.

Wistow, G. and B. Hardy. (1999). "The Development of Domiciliary Care: Mission Accomplished?" *Policy and Politics* 27 (2): 173-186.

Conclusions

"Home care, now more than ever." This was a headline in *The Globe and Mail* at the height of what we now know was the first outbreak of Severe Acute Respiratory Syndrome (SARS) in Toronto in the spring of 2003. The columnist, Jamie Swift, hailed home- and community-based care as the obvious panacea for a troubled public health system, one that is far too dependent on centralized hospital-based care. The failings of our current system of care could be better addressed, Swift believes, by enhancing home-based care. His model is the kind of care pioneered some 100 years ago by the Victorian Order of Nurses. These "women in starched, neatly-pressed uniforms" brought health care and home care to those in need. But as is well-known in some regions of Ontario, the VON today faces more challenges than attending to the care needs of individuals who have been released from hospital, or who are living with long-term health challenges in their homes. In some jurisdictions, the VON has been shut down, unable to provide care within a health care system that is more and more characterized by privatization and the incursion of the market system.

At the same time, in other jurisdictions such as Manitoba, the publicly funded and delivered home care system has much to commend, and may provide important lessons on how to build a better home care system for Canada as a whole. Considered pioneering at the time of its establishment in the 1970s, the Manitoba Continuing Care Program provides care that crosses community, hospital and nursing home boundaries; referral from any source (including self-referrals); short- and long-term community-based care without charge, based on need; public sector employees from a variety of disciplines to assess need and to provide services (staff in the program include professional nurses, social workers, physiotherapists, occupational therapists, as well as licensed practical nurses, home health aides, personal care workers, respite services and adult day care services); and a single-entry system linking assessed need for community care and need for nursing home admission (Shapiro 1997). Research on Manitoba's home care program shows that it has been able to provide integrated and comprehensive care at a lower cost than institutional care and does so for a large, and growing, number of individuals (Shapiro 1997). Moreover, Manitoba's home care program allows people to retain their independence and autonomy while affording them the comforts and security of home. As Armstrong and Armstrong (1996:136) observe, "Care in the home or 'community' is assumed to be better for virtually everyone and to be preferred by virtually everyone."

Of course, in Manitoba and other provinces with home care programs, there has been relatively little attention to the gendered nature of home care and unpaid caregiving, an issue that this collection of articles has shown to be a serious oversight. Home care and unpaid caregiving are issues for all Canadians, but especially so for women. As the majority of care providers and care recipients, the nature and availability of home care is a key issue for women. Whether they provide or receive care, women in Canada should have the right to care. In other words, those who need home care should be able to get that care in a form that is culturally appropriate and non-discriminatory, and those who provide it should not feel compelled to care such that their health, economic well-being and life opportunities are diminished (Charlottetown Declaration 2001).

The contention that home care is needed, "now more than ever," is a sentiment that has been repeated numerous times over the last several decades by many Canadians, including patients, caregivers, voluntary organizations, professional associations, policy analysts and researchers. The 1997 National Forum on Health called for a national home care program, and the recent Royal Commission on the Future of Health Care called for "a national platform for home care services," based on the recognition that "caregiving is becoming an increasing burden on many in our society, especially women" (Romanow 2002). To date, even in the face of mounting evidence of the value of home and community-based care, we continue to have a patchwork system of home care in Canada, and in most cases, we have a health care system that relies on family, friends and volunteers (many of whom are women) to provide care to those in need. No longer just a supplement to the health care system, many of those who provide care have become a substitute for a system under stress.

Throughout this book, the various contributors have demonstrated that caring matters – to those who provide care (whether they are paid or unpaid) and to those who receive (or would like to receive) care. And it especially matters to women because so much of the caring provided in this country is done by women, whether or not they are paid for this work. In recognizing that women's caring matters, we must make sure that the work is visible, valued and not taken for granted.

Home care and caregiving are essential services in the health care system today, particularly as health care reforms have meant an increasing shift of care from hospitals to the community and, more specifically, to individuals' homes. Whether the home is in fact the optimal site for care is often subordinated to the need to remove individuals from institutions. This presents challenges for caregivers and those cared for.

We have also seen that there are various segments of the population – whether identified on the basis of who they are, where they live or the state of their health – who find accessing and providing home care increasingly more difficult. The situation of Aboriginal Canadians and some who have disabilities perhaps best illustrates the gaps in our system. In Canada's rural and remote communities, the state of home and community-based care (not to mention institutional care) is particularly grave, as these areas have faced an increasing amount of de-population that has significantly affected the availability of formal health services, as well informal, family supports. Where issues of language and culture come into play, as is the case in Aboriginal communities, it becomes clear why we must think about care as a public, rather than simply private, issue.

Norah Keating has observed that the more individuals are involved in caring *for* people, the less time they have to care *about* people (Goldsand 1997). Of course, many of those involved in caregiving do care both for *and* about those in their care. The challenge is to imagine and make real a system that recognizes the rights, needs and aspirations of those receiving care, and of those providing care – whether or not they are being paid to provide that care. This means, as Nancy Guberman points out, building a care system based on principles of equity and justice. This also means, as Gillian Dalley (1988) has argued, thinking about care as not simply a personal matter between the caregiver and the recipient, but as a collective responsibility in our society.

The papers in this collection demonstrate that there is much that we already know about the needs of Canadians, and the demands on those who provide care. "Home care, now more than ever" makes sense. The real challenge is to build a home care system that works for women. When we have done that, we will have built a home care system that will benefit all Canadians.

References

Armstrong, P. and H. Armstrong. (1996). *Wasting Away: The Undermining of Canadian Health Care*. Toronto: Oxford University Press.

Charlottetown Declaration on the Right to Care. (2001). Charlottetown, PEI. Reprinted in A. Pederson and P. Beattie-Huggan (eds.), *The Objective is Care: Proceedings of The National Think Tank on Gender and Unpaid Caregiving* (2002), available at http://www.cewh-cesf.ca/healthreform/home_care/index.html

Dalley, G. (1988). *Ideologies of Caring: Rethinking Community and Collectivism*. London: Macmillan.

Goldsand, J. (1997). "Home Care Not Always the Best Care: What Governments Save Today May Cost Us Tomorrow." *University of Alberta Folio*, 21 March. Online at http://www.ualberta.ca/~publicas/folio/34/14/04.html

Romanow, R. (2002). *Building on Values: The Future of Health Care in Canada – Final Report*. Ottawa: The Royal Commission on the Future of Health Care in Canada.

Shapiro, E. (1997). *The Cost of Privatization: A Case Study of Home Care in Manitoba*. Ottawa: Canadian Centre for Policy Alternatives.

Swift, J. (2003). "Home Care, Now More Than Ever." *The Globe and Mail*, April 24, A15.

About the Contributors

The editors of this volume make up the current and one former member of The National Coordinating Group on Health Care Reform and Women. We are:

- Karen R. Grant (Department of Sociology, University of Manitoba), member from the National Network on Environments and Women's Health).
- Pat Armstrong (see below). Chair, and member of the National Network on Environments and Women's Health.
- Carol Amaratunga (Ontario Women's Health Council/University of Ottawa Chair in Women's Health), former member from the Atlantic Centre of Excellence for Women's Health.
- Madeline Boscoe, member from the Canadian Women's Health Network.
- Ann Pederson, member from the British Columbia Centre of Excellence for Women's Health.
- Kay Willson, member from the Prairie Women's Health Centre of Excellence.

CONTRIBUTORS TO THIS VOLUME:

Pat Armstrong is a Professor of Sociology at Toronto's York University and holder of a Canadian Health Services Research/Canadian Institutes of Health Research Chair in health policy and women. She has published numerous books and articles on women's work, pay equity and health care policy in Canada.

Hugh Armstrong is a Professor of Social Work at Carleton University in Ottawa. He has published eight books and numerous articles focusing on health care policy, the political economy of health, women and work, and unions and public policy.

Jane Aronson is a Professor of Social Work at McMaster University in Hamilton. She specializes in the study of women, aging, caring work, and health.

Nancy Guberman is a Professor of Social Work at L'Université du Québec à Montréal. Her research focuses on women's work, family caregiving, and the women's movement in Quebec.

Erika Haug is an instructor with the Indian Social Work program at the First Nations University of Canada (formerly Saskatchewan Indian Federated College) in Saskatoon.

Michelle Hogan is a mixed-blood Anishinabe woman from Batchewana First Nation, currently in her fourth Year of Indian Studies, who has also been a home care recipient.

Olga Kits is a policy analyst with the Ontario Ministry of Health in Toronto and has worked on the regulation of health professions and the medical errors/ patient safety portfolio; she has an MA from Queen's University.

Kari Krogh is a CIHR Senior Research Fellow in the School of Disability Studies at Ryerson University. She is a disability activist and academic specializing in emancipatory research methods including participatory health policy analysis.

Jason McCarthy is a third-year Métis social work student at the First Nations University of Canada (formerly Saskatchewan Indian Federated College).

Lorraine MacDonald is a member of Smith's Landing First Nation, Northwest Territories, who has fifteen years experience in social work, community and economic development with the federal, territorial and First Nations governments.

Marika Morris is Research Coordinator of CRIAW. She is the author of a number of papers and publications on women's health, poverty and gender-based analyses of public policies. She is completing her doctorate at Carleton University.

Shelley Thomas Prokop is a member of Beardy's and Okemasis First Nation in Saskatchewan and an Assistant professor with the Indian Social Work program at the First Nations University of Canada (formerly Saskatchewan Indian Federated College) in Saskatoon.

Index

Métis people 102
minimum wage 14, 16
and women 108
minority groups
and access to health care 29
and barriers to care 101
and discrimination 106
and privatization 18
and rural care 33
mobility rights 138
models of disability 117-18
multiple care recipients 94
multiple sclerosis care recipients 51

NAFTA, *see* North American Free Trade Agreement 14
nation state
end of 14
power of 14
National Advisory Council on Aging 153
National Forum on Health 48, 65
National Population Health Survey (NPHS) 92, 94
national sovereignty and globalization 14
National standard for home care 138, 139, 167
National Think Tank on Gender and Unpaid Caregiving 1
Native Women's Association of Canada (NWAC) 155
Native, *see* Aboriginal women
natural caregivers 9, 24, 78, 106
neglect, *see* abuse
negotiating home care 179
Neysmith, Sheila 82
NGOs, *see* Non-Governmental Organizations
nonapparent impairments, perceptions of 120-21
Non-Governmental Organizations
and funding 22
and provision of care 21-22
and role of women 22
North American Free Trade Agreement and public health care 14
NWAC, *see* Native Women's Association of Canada

obligation to care 24, 54, 59, 64, 103

"enforced altruism" 176
and gender division 81
Old Age Pension 61
Oliver, Michael 129
Ontario and home care 169
Ontario case study on reorganization of health care 169
oppression and disability 123
options for care 77-78
see also choice
organization of care 47-48

pain limitations and gender 121, 122
palliative care 48, 53
parents as caregivers, stress on 99
Parkinson's disease
and effects on caregivers 108
patients and impact on caregivers 55
participation of care recipients in health care system 85
Participation and Activity Limitation Survey 122
partner, *see* spouses
patients as caregivers 92
peer support and self-directed care 132
pension
rights 15, 59
schemes and the welfare state 61, 62
perceptions
of disability 119
of impairments 131
personal assistance and home care 115
politics, body 9, 118–19, 130
poverty 58
and Aboriginal peoples 153
power
and community care 32
and consumers 20
distribution of 9-10
in the workplace 28
dynamics of knowledge 161
and economic status 12
gaps in 18
relationships 38
practical needs of disabled people 85
preventative measures and training 86
prevention, disease 30, 62, 85
Prince Edward Island, disability-supports program 136

privacy
and informal caring 56
loss of in household 56
and the state 25
Trudeau 25
private care
costs of 22
impact on women 27
privatization
of health services and impact on Aboriginal women 158
impact on home care and women 125
impact on women and work 17
and minority groups 18
professionalization of care 161
profile of a caregiver 51, 86-87, 95
spouses as caregivers 53
friends as caregivers 54
property rights and women 17
protection
for care recipients 126
lack of for caregivers 100
provincial
differences in support networks 60
responsibility for home care 138
provision of health care on reserves 154-55
public care
vs. family care 8
reforms in 21
and North American Free Trade Agreement 14
public sector
definition of care 27-28
employment protections 25
expansion of 25
and privatization 17
and unions 25
Public Service Alliance of Canada 50
public services, impact of decline 12

quality of care 82, 172, 174-75
and cost-cutting 125
and efficiency 133
financial influences 92
influences on 84

race and diabetes 13
racism
and Aboriginals 148, 154